PRACTICAL HEAD & NECK ULTRASOUND

PRACTICAL HEAD & NECK ULTRASOUND

Edited by

Anil T Ahuja

MBBS (Bombay) MD (Bombay) FRCR
  FHKCR FHKAM

Associate Professor
Department of Diagnostic
Radiology and Organ Imaging
Chinese University of Hong Kong
Prince of Wales Hospital
Shatin
Hong Kong
China

Rhodri M Evans

MB BCh FRCR

Consultant Radiologist
Radiology Department
Morriston Hospital
Morriston
Swansea
Wales
UK

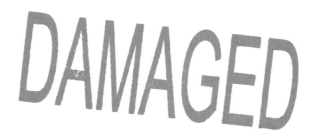

CAMBRIDGE UNIVERSITY PRESS
Cambridge, New York, Melbourne, Madrid, Cape Town, Singapore, São Paulo

CAMBRIDGE UNIVERSITY PRESS
The Edinburgh Building, Cambridge CB2 2RU, UK

Published in the United States of America by Cambridge University Press, New York

www.cambridge.org
Information on this title: www.cambridge.org/9780521683210

First published 2000
Reprinted by Cambridge University Press 2006

Printed in the United Kingdom at the University Press, Cambridge

A catalogue record for this publication is available from the British Library

ISBN-13 978-0-521-683210 paperback
ISBN-10 0-521-683211 paperback

CONTENTS

CHAPTER 1

Anatomy and Technique *R M Evans*

CHAPTER 2

Salivary Glands *M J Bradley*

CHAPTER 3

The Thyroid and Parathyroids *A T Ahuja*

CHAPTER 4

Lymph Nodes *R M Evans*

CHAPTER 5

Lumps and Bumps in the Head and Neck *A T Ahuja*

CHAPTER 6

The Larynx *E Loveday*

CHAPTER 7

What the Surgeon Needs to Know, and Why *D W Patton, K C Silvester*

CHAPTER 8

CHAPTER 9

CONTRIBUTORS

Anil T Ahuja MBBS (Bom) MD (Bom)
FRCR FHKCR FHKAM
Associate Professor
Department of Diagnostic Radiology and
Organ Imaging
Chinese University of Hong Kong
Prince of Wales Hospital
Shatin, Hong Kong
China

Laurence Berman FRCP FRCR
Consultant Radiologist Lecturer/Honorary Consultant
University Department of Radiology
Addenbrooke's Hospital NHS Trust
Hills Road
Cambridge

Michael Jameson Bradley MB BCH FRCR
Consultant Radiologist and Honorary Senior
Clinical Lecturer
X Ray Department
North Bristol Trust
Southmead Hospital
Westbury-on-Trym
Bristol, UK

Neil Cozens DMRD FRCR
Consultant Radiologist
Derbyshire Royal Infirmary NHS Trust
Derby, UK

Rhodri M Evans MB BCh FRCR
Consultant Radiologist
Radiology Department
Morriston Hospital
Morriston, Swansea
Wales, UK

Stella S Y Ho MPhil RDMS RVT
Senior Radiographer
Department of Diagnostic Radiology and Organ Imaging
Chinese University of Hong Kong
Prince of Wales Hospital
Shatin, Hong Kong
China

Eric Loveday
Consultant Radiologist
X Ray Department
Southmead Hospital
Westbury-on-Trym
Bristol, UK

C Metreweli FRCR FRCP
Professor and Chairman
Department of Diagnostic Radiology and Organ Imaging
Chinese University of Hong Kong
Prince of Wales Hospital
Shatin, Hong Kong
China

David William Patton TD FDS FRCS
Consultant Oral and Maxillofacial Surgeon
Department of Oral and Maxillofacial Surgery
Morriston Hospital
Morriston, Swansea
Wales, UK

Keith Charles Silvester MBBS (Lond) BDS (Lond)
FDS RCS (Eng) FRCS (Ed)
Consultant Oral and Facial Surgeon
Department of Oral and Maxillofacial Surgery
Morriston Hospital
Morriston, Swansea
Wales, UK

INTRODUCTION

We have the privilege of working and living during a time of unprecedented technological advances in diagnostic medicine. This now means that for any one diagnostic problem we have not only have one method of imaging but many methods available to us. Wise use of the various technologies dictates that the most informative, least harmful, most easily available and least expensive techniques should be employed first.

With the arrival of CT, MRI, ultrasound and nuclear medicine in medical imaging, a new era of diagnostic understanding of the head and neck has flowered.

In the soft tissues of the neck, many of the diagnostic problems that present to the clinician can be managed with maximal efficiency using ultrasound. Surprisingly, despite the pioneering of neck ultrasound by Bruneton and Solbiati, a large number of neck examinations are still being performed using nuclear medicine, CT and MRI. One might have thought that neck ultrasound would thrive in hospitals in which CT and, particularly, MRI are not readily available. Alas, it seems that most clinicians would prefer to let their patients wait several weeks for MRI and then not get a satisfactory answer, rather than obtain an ultrasound scan quickly from a knowledgeable professional and have an accurate answer sooner.

There are several texts on imaging of the head and neck[1,2] but these are predominantly CT and MRI orientated. Apart from chapters in Solbiati and Rizzatto's book,[3] there is very little helpful information to enable the radiologist in a busy general hospital to come to grips with ultrasound of the head and neck. This is unfortunate – quite apart from the usual well-known advantages of ultrasound in the head and neck, it is remarkably accurate and easier to apply than CT and MRI.

This book therefore aims to fill that gap. The text is intended as a practical guide and bench book. It is to be hoped that it will encourage anyone with a reasonable knowledge of ultrasound to pick up the (appropriate!) transducer and start scanning the neck effectively rather than simply 'gel spreading'. It is intended to help the reader to be able to reach a useful opinion in 90% of the problems that arise in daily practice. The remaining 10% will have to be learnt from personal experience and greater in-depth reading. By the Paredo principle, trying to cover that 10% would probably quadruple the size of this book, so do not expect this book to have the answer to everything.

Besides omitting rarities we have also avoided myths – those anecdotal 'facts' that keep reappearing in textbooks and examinations but which one never sees in daily practice.

The book contains the sort of information that we wish we could have had when we started neck scanning ten years ago. Much of the information is available in the literature but is scattered. Here the most useful information is gathered together by people who actually scan; the 'litter-ature' has therefore been weeded out.

Please note that this book is intended for those who will actually scan. It depends on an interactive approach. It is not meant for the CPR (couch potato radiologist) who sits back and lets others perform the scan and then 'reports the films!'. We strongly believe that this is not the way to practice ultrasound. We are also strong believers in the opinion that (good) ultrasound is not 'operator dependent', at least no more so than MRI, CT or, for that matter, surgery or pathology. The claim that ultrasound is operator dependent is merely a feeble line of defence for CPRs who are unwilling to roll up their sleeves and learn how to do the job properly!

For thyroid nodules, we can now make a diagnosis with ultrasound that can be more reliable than fine-needle aspiration cytology (FNAC) and far more useful than scintigraphy, which surprisingly is still mentioned in the texts as being a method of choice. It is high time that thyroid scintigraphy took its proper place – in the history books, alongside air encephalography.

With neck lymph nodes we can now examine their vascularity, not only with colour flow and power Doppler but also with 3D volumetric analysis. The detail that can be seen in lymph nodes is superior to and more clinically useful than that obtained by either CT or MRI.

The characterisation and localisation of salivary gland tumours is simple and easy without the need to inject contrast or cannulate the ducts. Even those mysterious lumps and bumps that do not seem to belong to the expected organs reveal their secrets to ultrasound.

In many cases one is able to make a confident diagnosis before FNAC or histology, but in those cases where this is still indicated ultrasound is the imaging technique of choice in guiding the needle to its best target. Palpation-guided FNA is not only barbaric but inaccurate. Those who know how difficult it is to guide a needle into a target under direct visual control will know why the blind approach is inaccurate. In these days 'blind' biopsy 'technique' must surely mean 'blind to the benefits of guided biopsy'.

Lest the reader consider this book too dogmatic, we appreciate that there are still major controversies to sort out, and different centres have varying strengths and therefore different approaches to diagnostic management .This is best exemplified by the chapter dealing with biopsy techniques which voices the different approaches that can be used in the head and neck.

Despite its multiple authorship this book has a feeling of common purpose and I would like to think, with considerable pride, that this is the result of a common origin for several of the authors. Rhodri Evans, Mike Bradley and Eric Loveday have all passed through my department in the Chinese University of Hong Kong at the Prince of Wales Hospital. It was here that they learnt the initial skills and have been able to take these back to Europe (I believe that Britain is considered, by some, to be part of Europe in a peripheral sort of way!) and to develop them further.

Most of the authors have taught at the Morriston Head and Neck Ultrasound Workshops. As the Morriston course evolved, it became clear that there is a real need for a co-ordinated approach to the head and neck. This text should fill that need. The spectrum of topics discussed should provide the necessary background for anyone starting out in head and neck ultrasound.

The Morriston course has not so far not included a section on carotid and vertebral ultrasound/Doppler; however, it was felt that this is an essential component of neck ultrasound and has therefore been added. The sonologist or sonographer who deals with the head and neck must be competent not only in grey-scale ultrasound but colour flow and pulsed Doppler as well. In the neck we have the opportunity of using every new technique that the ultrasound designers can give us!

It is gratifying to learn that the European Association of Radiology has now recognised head and neck imaging as a subspecialty in its own right, alongside such older worthies as neuroradiology and paediatric radiology.

This handbook is therefore timely and we hope that it will add a small, but useful, gust to the necessary winds of change.

Con Metreweli

References

1. Som PM, Curtin HD. *Head and Neck Imaging,* 3rd edn. St Louis: Mosby–Year Book, 1996.

2. Harnsberger HR. *Handbook of Head and Neck Imaging,* 2nd edn. St Louis: Mosby–Year Book, 1995.

3. Solbiati L, Rizzatto G. *Ultrasound of Superficial Structures.* Edinburgh: Churchill Livingstone, 1995.

ACKNOWLEDGEMENT

This text is the result of a team effort. We therefore say 'thank you' to the team. We would particularly like to thank 'Prof M' for giving us both the opportunity to develop our interest in head and neck ultrasound. We also owe a large debt of gratitude to our colleagues and staff of our respective hospitals, namely: The Prince of Wales Hospital, Shatin, Hong Kong; Morriston Hospital, Swansea and Neath General Hospital for their generous support, not just in the writing and editing of this text but also in the organising and running of the Morriston Workshops.

On a more personal level we must acknowledge the close support and help provided by our families. For Anil this is, in particular, his wife Chu Wai Po, his mother and his late father. On Rhodri's part – 'Diolch yn fawr i Lynne, Catrin, Bethan a Gwyn'.

Anil and Rhodri

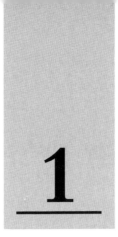

1

ANATOMY AND TECHNIQUE

RM Evans

Equipment and technique
Anatomy: introduction
Ultrasound anatomy

Introduction

Over the past two decades, rapid strides in ultrasound (US) technology and in particular the development of high resolution US have led to a greater role for ultrasound in the assessment of the extracranial head and neck. The increased spatial resolution achieved by the latest generation of machines and transducers allows excellent near field resolution. When one considers that the majority of structures and associated pathology in the neck lie only between one and five centimetres below the skin surface, and given the superior resolution that high resolution US can attain, it is not surprising that US is gaining in popularity in the field of head and neck imaging. As it is relatively inexpensive (in Radiology terms) and is readily available, the use of US will continue to increase.

One criticism of US is that it is 'operator dependent'. While there can be no argument with that statement, it is not a criticism that is made of other imaging techniques, which are equally operator dependent. We accept that cytology is operator dependent, we know that surgery is operator dependent, so why is 'operator dependent' a criticism that is continually heard when US is discussed? Most medicine is operator dependent in one form or other; the myth that US is more 'operator dependent' than other techniques should be laid to rest. If one is enthusiastic and willing to learn, the learning curve in US is no steeper than that in magnetic resonance imaging (MRI), computed tomography (CT), or any other branch of radiology.

The key to an understanding of the neck, as in all other areas of radiology, is a sound knowledge of anatomy. The aim of this chapter is to provide that knowledge as a basis for understanding ultrasound of the neck.

Equipment and technique

A state-of-the-art high resolution US machine is desirable but not essential. A dedicated high resolution US machine is a luxury for most of those who work in busy US departments; however, most reputable multifunction machines now have sufficient high resolution hardware, software and probes to allow adequate examination of the head and neck. A linear 7.5–10 MHz probe with a relatively small 'footprint', i.e. a small contact surface area, is optimal. Higher frequency probes, i.e. 10 MHz and above, allow superior resolution for superficial structures but there is a trade-off in lack of depth penetration. Be aware that a probe of too high a

frequency, i.e. 10–13 MHz, can definitely be counterproductive when learning; for the beginner, an appreciation of the overall anatomy is much more easily obtained using lower frequency probes. There is a role for 5 MHz probes in assessing deep lesions such as those in the deep lobe of the parotid. Colour flow facilities are now standard on most machines; and while preferable they are not necessarily essential. The beginner will find it easier to pick out the vascular anatomy of the neck using colour flow, but there will be less dependence once familiarity with the anatomy has been attained. Power flow applications are desirable for assessing flow patterns, for example in lymph nodes and thyroid nodules. The beginner may be deterred from carrying out a biopsy in the head and neck if colour imaging is regularly used. Many head and neck tumours and lymph nodes have spectacular colour flow features but core biopsy and fine-needle aspiration biopsy (FNAB) can still be safely carried out!

One essential piece of equipment is a high quality, adjustable and mobile table. It is important that for US and US guided procedures in the neck, the examiner is comfortable. A mobile table that can be easily positioned so that the patient's neck is level with the US monitor and within the operators scanning range is essential. Most operators find the most comfortable position to be, one in which the patient's neck is level with the examiner's thigh or knees. When carrying out biopsy techniques the operator must be positioned so that the monitor can be viewed comfortably without undue stretching or twisting. A monitor on a manoeuvrable arm is ideal. The patient's neck should be sufficiently close so that both the hand holding the probe and the hand holding the needle or biopsy gun are in a relaxed position, again without undue stretching or twisting. The probe, needle, monitor and patient should be in a tight or acute field of view for optimal positioning. Comfort of operator and patient will reduce problems when free-hand biopsies are performed under real-time US control. While this appears to be no more common sense, most of the problems encountered by the author when teaching free-hand biopsy techniques are due to poor positioning of both radiologist and patient.

The patient should be positioned with the neck extended, a pillow behind the shoulders and lower neck allowing the patient to adopt a comfortable position that can be maintained throughout the study. There may be difficulties in elderly patients with arthritic necks or respiratory problems; in these patients the table should be adjusted to 45 degrees and a pillow placed behind the shoulders, if possible, to enable some extension of the neck. The patient may be scanned in a sitting position if necessary, although assessment of the lower neck may be compromised.

The use of a gel block is sometimes required, particularly if one is not blessed with a probe with a small footprint. Integrated stand-off blocks are not necessary. In certain 'angular' positions, such as the angle of the mandible and supraclavicular fossa in thin individuals, a better image will be obtained using a stand off block. The author finds a small (9 cm), round gel disc (Aqua flex gel pad, Parker laboratories, USA) to be the most satisfactory. It is washable and usually lasts for 4–6 weeks in a busy department. If one has a high frequency probe with a small footprint, the application of a good covering of gel is usually sufficient for the assessment of the most superficial structures.

Anatomy: introduction

As in any field of radiology, an understanding of the anatomy of the region is the key to the radiological approach. Unfortunately the complex anatomy of the

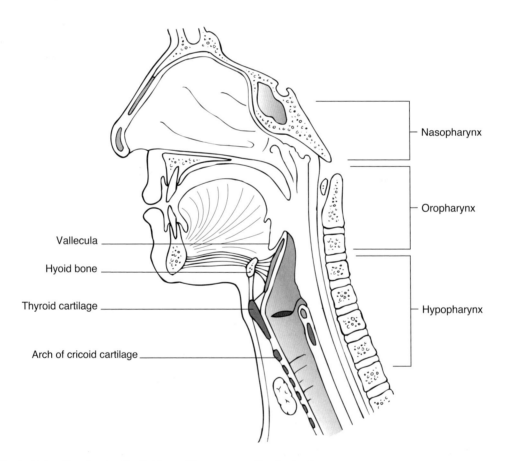

Nasopharynx

Oropharynx

Hypopharynx

Vallecula

Hyoid bone

Thyroid cartilage

Arch of cricoid cartilage

Figure 1.1 – Sagittal section showing the divisions of the upper aerodigestive tract.

head and neck can prove a daunting prospect for the radiologist who only infrequently carries out scanning in this area. The situation is not helped by the many and varied methods and concepts employed in describing the anatomy of the extracranial head and neck.

Traditionally, the upper aerodigestive tract is divided into four areas: nasopharynx, oropharynx, hypopharynx and oral cavity. These subdivisions are important in CT and MRI but of less significance in ultrasound. All radiologists should be aware of these traditional divisions (Figure 1.1). They are relevant in the diagnosis and staging of squamous cell carcinoma (SCC), the most prevalent tumour of the upper aerodigestive tract.[1]

Surgeons and anatomists[2] have traditionally divided the neck into triangles based on muscular landmarks and boundaries. This division of the neck into triangles does not sit easily with the cross-sectional anatomy techniques practised by radiologists, however radiologists must be aware of the surgical system in order to comprehend referrals for imaging (Figure 1.2).

Knowledge of the anatomy of just three muscles – the sternocleidomastoid, digastric and omohyoid – is the key to understanding the triangles of the neck. The sternocleidomastoid, which runs from the mastoid process to the clavicle and sternum, divides the neck into two large triangles: anterior and posterior.

The anterior triangle is subdivided into supra- and infra-hyoid portions. The suprahyoid portion is further divided by the anterior belly of digastric muscle into the submental and submandibular triangles. The infrahyoid portion is divided by the superior belly of the omohyoid muscle into muscular and carotid triangles. The posterior belly of digastric marks the superior border of the carotid triangle.

The posterior triangle is demarcated by the posterior border of sternomastoid anteriorly and the anterior border of trapezius posteriorly. The apex is formed by the occiput while the base of the triangle is formed by the clavicle. The triangle is further subdivided by the posterior belly of the omohyoid muscle, forming an occipital triangle superiorly and a supraclavicular triangle inferiorly. The division of the neck by the sternomastoid often poses a dilemma in that a mass deep to the sternomastoid is not strictly in the anterior or the posterior triangle, the posterior border of sternomas-

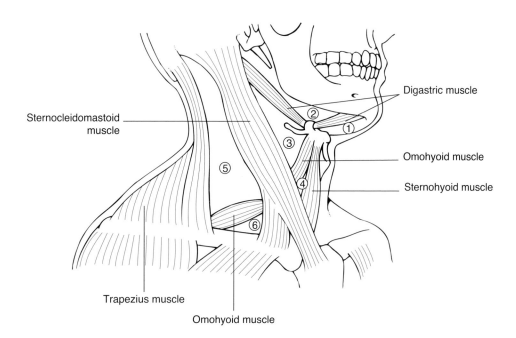

Figure 1.2 – Division of the neck into 'triangles'. The anterior triangle is divided into ① submental ② submandibular, ③ carotid and ④ muscular triangles. The posterior triangle is divided into a ⑤ occipital triangle and an ⑥ supraclavicular.

toid demarcating the anterior boundary of the posterior triangle.

The advent of CT and MRI has brought about a reappraisal by radiologists of the anatomy of the extracranial head and neck. The multiplanar capabilities of MRI in particular have enabled a far better appreciation of the complex anatomy of this region. The 'spaces' concept has been heralded as the key to a better understanding of the anatomy and pathology of the head and neck. Radiologists, in particular Harnsberger,[3-6] have developed a clear and practical method of using the spaces concept to analyse head and neck pathology (Figures 1.3, 1.4). Above the hyoid bone the spaces concept works well and knowledge of the suprahyoid spaces aids assessment with ultrasound, however the same is not true when assessing the infrahyoid neck.

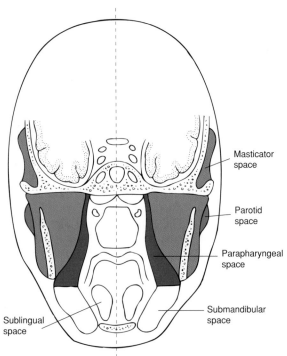

Figure 1.4 – Coronal section showing the major spaces. Note the cranial/caudal extension of the parapharyngeal and masticator spaces. Note also the communication between the parapharyngeal and submandibular spaces.

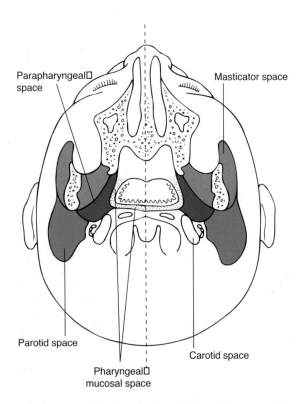

Figure 1.3 – Axial section depicting the 'big five' spaces of the neck, i.e. parapharyngeal space (red), parotid space (blue), carotid space, masticator space (brown), and pharyngeal mucosal space.

Ultrasound anatomy

'Where do I start?' is a familiar plea when attempting ultrasound of the head and neck. It is essential to have an easily replicated systematic strategy for the examination of the extracranial head and neck. This allows key structures to be identified and enables assessment of the whole neck. The aim of this chapter is to present a strategy that allows the sonographer or radiologist to quickly and systematically examine the neck.

The ensuing method follows a logical progression from mandible to clavicle in direction. For each region the key structures that can be, and need to be, identified will be highlighted.

Submental region (Figure 1.5)

The borders of the submental triangle are easily defined on ultrasound. The floor is formed by the mylohyoid muscle, and the apex of the triangle by the symphysis mentis, the base of the triangle being formed by the hyoid bone. The anterior belly of the digastric muscles represent the sides of the triangle. These can be followed down in transverse section to the hyoid. The only contents of note are the submental lymph node group.

The genioglossus and geniohyoid muscles form the root of the tongue. Together with the hyoglossus muscle they make up the major extrinsic muscles of the tongue. The mylohyoid muscle is synonymous with the floor of mouth, forming a muscular sling between the medial aspect of the mandibular bodies. Posteriorly the mylohyoid has a free thick border and is thinner anteriorly where it is attached to the anterior mandible inferior to the origins of the genial muscles (genioglossus and geniohyoid). The anterior portion of the mylohyoid can be difficult to demonstrate, and in some instances it is deficient anteriorly.

The lingual artery can be easily picked up using colour flow imaging, and is a readily recognised landmark. It is just medial to the hyoglossus muscle. Differentiation between the mylohyoid and hyoglossus muscles can be aided by scanning in the coronal plane, while asking the patient to move the tongue from side to side. The mylohyoid is relatively immobile while the hyoglossus

is identified actively contracting (see Figure 1.6b, c). Contraction of the hyoglossus muscle depresses the tongue. Lateral to the hyoglossus, the submandibular duct can be identified[7], particularly if it is dilated (see Figure 1.6d). Take care not to confuse the duct with the lingual vein which sits alongside the proximal submandibular duct; colour flow imaging usually identifies the vein. The submandibular duct is sandwiched with the sublingual gland between the hyoglossus and mylohyoid muscles. It lies just superior and lateral to the lingual artery, which can be identified medial to the hyoglossus muscle (Fig 1.6b).

The sublingual gland is identified on transverse or axial sections as an elongated hyperechoic structure, lateral to hyoglossus. It is much larger than is generally appreciated: anteriorly it almost touches the symphysis mentis and posteriorly it abuts the deep surface of the submandibular gland. The submandibular duct often receives a large accessory duct from the anterior part of the sublingual gland (Bartholin's duct). The sublingual gland may be joined to the submandibular gland to form a large, single sublingual–submandibular complex.

The mylohyoid muscle is the key to differentiating whether or not a lesion is in the sublingual or submandibular space. Lesions deep to mylohyoid are within the sublingual space; if a lesion is superficial to mylohyoid it lies within the submandibular space (see Figure 1.4). Around the posterior border of the mylo-

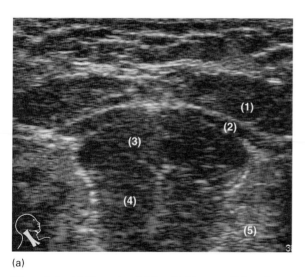

(a)

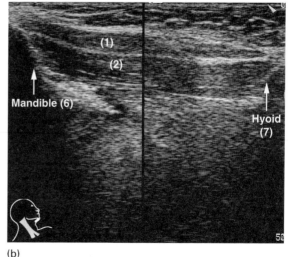

(b)

Figure 1.5 – (a) Coronal and (b) sagittal images of the submental region. (1) Anterior belly of digastric muscle. (2) Mylohyoid. (3) Geniohyoid. (4) Genioglossus. (5) Sublingual gland. (6) Mandible. (7) Hyoid.

hyoid muscle free communication is possible between the posterior sublingual space and the adjacent submandibular and inferior parapharyngeal space (as in a diving ranula – a retention cyst of the sublingual gland that extends posteriorly into the submandibular space and inferiorly into the parapharyngeal space).

The submandibular duct extends anteriorly from the gland within the submandibular space into the sublingual space, swerving around the free posterior border of mylohyoid.

Submandibular region (Figure 1.6)

The submandibular gland sits like a saddle astride the digastric and mylohyoid muscles when viewed in a transverse plane. The anterior belly of the digastric may be seen emerging anteriorly. The anterior belly of the digastric is more muscular and easier to define than the tendinous portion of the posterior belly which is identified immediately posterior to the body of the submandibular gland. The tendon of the posterior belly can be followed down towards the hyoid. Immediately

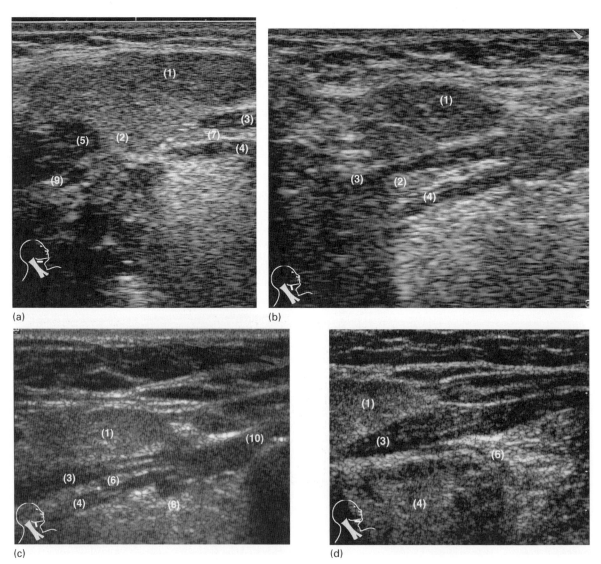

(a) (b)

(c) (d)

Figure 1.6 – (a) Transverse, (b) coronal, (c) coronal oblique, (d) transverse views of the submandibular region. (1) Superficial submandibular gland. (2) Deep submandibular gland. (3) Mylohyoid. (4) Hyoglossus. (5) Posterior belly of digastric. (6) Submandibular duct. (7) Lingual vein. (8) Lingual artery. (9) Facial artery. (10) Hyoid.

inferior to the submandibular gland it cannot usually be seen as it splits the stylohyoid muscle and then enters its fascial tunnel. The submandibular gland lies in the plane of the anterior belly of digastric, hence more of the anterior belly is identified in parasagittal sections of the submandibular gland than the posterior belly which runs in a more cranial–caudal orientation, i.e. more vertically. More posteriorly the mylohyoid is visible, its posterior free border indenting the submandibular gland.

Anterior to the submandibular gland is a small, fat-filled triangular space. Lymph nodes can be identified in this region. Two constant venous landmarks outline the submandibular gland; anteriorly and superiorly the facial vein can be seen coursing superficially, and posteriorly the anterior division of the retromandibular vein can be identified. This joins with the facial vein to drain into the internal jugular vein. Displacement of this venous structure is the key to differentiating whether a mass is arising from the submandibular gland anteriorly or the parotid gland posteriorly. The superficial venous anatomy of the neck, while variable, provides many recognisable landmarks (Figure 1.7). The serpiginous course of the facial artery can be identified

with colour flow imaging as it passes deep to the anterior portion of the submandibular gland. It emerges from behind the mid/anterior portion of the gland to pass up and over the body of mandible.

Parotid region (Figure 1.8)

The parotid space extends from the external auditory meatus superiorly to the angle of the mandible inferiorly. Within the gland lies the retromandibular vein (RMV) and, just medial to it, the external carotid artery (ECA). The RMV is a landmark for the facial nerve which courses just laterally. The RMV can be taken as a marker for the division of the parotid into superficial and deep lobes. Alternatively, an imaginary line drawn along the axis of the ramus of the mandible through the parotid acts to divide the superficial and deep lobes. The main parotid duct is identified as an echogenic line within the superficial lobe. The masseter muscle lies just deep to the anterior aspect of the superficial lobe, and accessory lobes of the parotid are identified in this region. The parotid duct runs approximately one finger breadth below the zygomatic arch, coursing anteriorly through the buccal space before

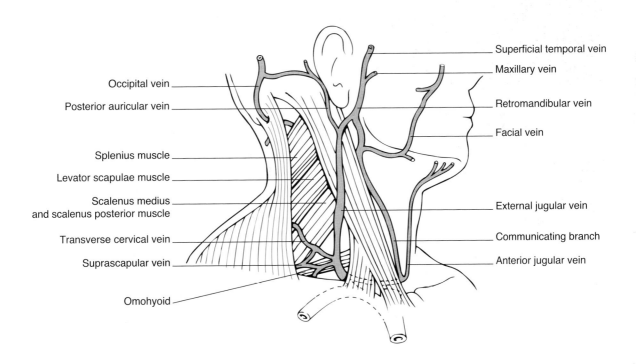

Figure 1.7 – Superficial venous anatomy of the neck.

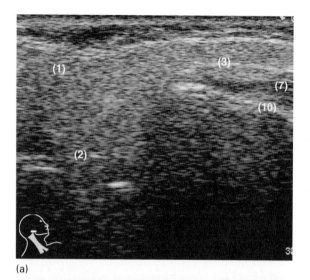

(a)

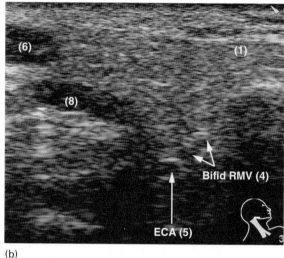

Bifid RMV (4)

ECA (5)

(b)

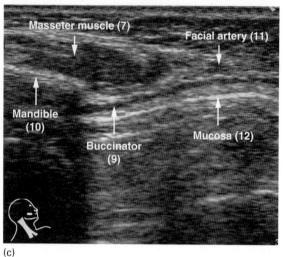

Masseter muscle (7)

Facial artery (11)

Mandible
(10)

Buccinator
(9)

Mucosa (12)

(c)

Figure 1.8 – (a) Axial image of body of parotid, (b) axial image of parotid tail, (c) axial image of buccal region. (1) Superficial lobe parotid. (2) Deep lobe parotid. (3) Parotid duct. (4) Retromandibular vein. (5) External carotid artery. (6) Sternomastoid. (7) Masseter. (8) Posterior belly digastric. (9) Buccinator. (10) Mandible. (11) Facial artery. (12) Mucosa.

piercing the buccinator muscle. The thin buccinator muscle extends anteriorly and just medially to the anterior margin of the masseter (Figure 1.8c). Asking the patient to blow out the cheek or clench the teeth aids its identification. The buccal space, which lies lateral to the buccinator muscle, contains fat, the facial nerve, vein, artery and parotid duct.

Upper cervical region (Figure 1.9)

As the probe passes down from the tail of the parotid gland the operator is confronted by a minefield of vascular structures. Colour flow imaging is of great assistance in this area.

The two structures to pick out are the internal jugular vein (IJV), which acts as the landmark for the deep cervical lymph node chain, and the posterior belly of digastric muscle. The posterior belly of the digastric muscle is a key structure in separating the parotid region from the upper cervical region inferiorly. Clinically, the posterior belly of the digastric muscle marks the division between the submandibular triangle anteriorly and the carotid triangle more posteriorly. To identify it, align the probe just anterior to the mastoid process, directing down towards the hyoid. The posterior belly of digastric will be identified emerging deep to sternomastoid muscle to abut the tail of the parotid. It is a superficial structure and courses at approximately

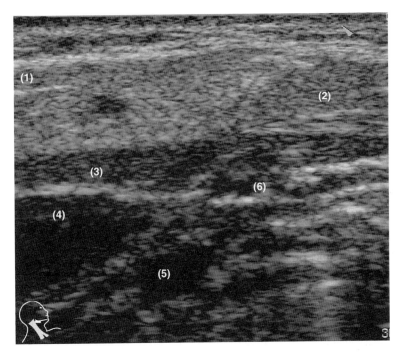

Figure 1.9 – Axial image of the upper cervical region. (1) Parotid gland. (2) Submandibular gland. (3) Posterior belly digastric. (4) Internal jugular vein. (5) Internal carotid artery. (6) External carotid artery. Note the union of the parotid and submandibular glands (normal variant).

45 degrees to the plane of the north–south axis of the parotid gland; the retromandibular vein and its connection to the external jugular vein can be seen passing superficial to it. This is the only major vascular structure that is superficial to the posterior belly of digastric.

By turning the probe slightly inferiorly along the line of the posterior belly of digastric the vessels deep to it are seen. From posterior to anterior, they are the internal jugular vein, internal carotid artery and external carotid artery (Figure 1.10).

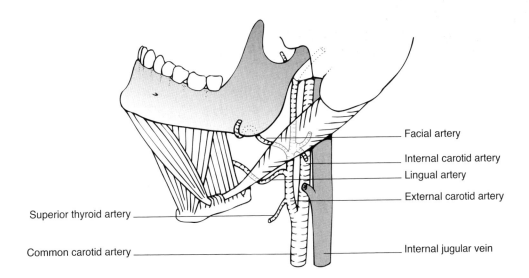

Figure 1.10 – The key relationships of the posterior belly of digastric muscle.

In thin necks the transverse process of the atlas may be identified, situated halfway between the mastoid process and the angle of the mandible.

Mid cervical region (Figure 1.11)

Where does the upper cervical region end and the mid cervical region begin? The cervical region is divided into upper and mid portions by the hyoid bone. The cricoid cartilage divides mid from lower portions.

The omohyoid muscle is an important surgical landmark. The superior belly of omohyoid divides the infrahyoid portion of the anterior triangle into carotid and muscular triangles whilst the posterior or inferior belly divides the posterior triangle into occipital and subclavian triangles. Many tumours are treated by tumour resection with a supra-omohyoid lymph node dissection. The omohyoid also represents an important landmark in the radical neck dissection.

The omohyoid arises from the anterior portion of the body of the hyoid bone before running obliquely to cross anterior to the common carotid artery and then deep to sternomastoid. It has an intermediate tendon which passes through a fascial sling attached to the clavicle. At this point it occasionally overlies the IJV but is usually found immediately lateral to it, where it may be mistaken for a lymph node. It then runs obliquely again across the fascial carpet of the inferior posterior triangle to attach to the posterior aspect of the lateral clavicle.

The key structures of the mid cervical region are the common carotid artery (CCA) and IJV. Scanning inferiorly in a transverse plane detects any adjacent lymph nodes and allows the omohyoid to be identified crossing from medial to lateral over the CCA. This point is usually at the level of the cricoid cartilage, demarcating the division between the mid and lower portions of the deep cervical chain. When scanning transversely, just

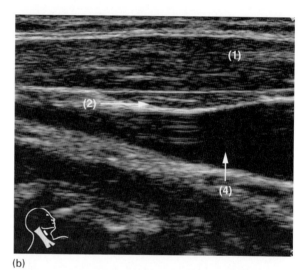

(b)

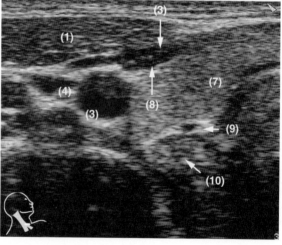

(a)

(c)

Figure 1.11 – (a) Axial and (b) sagittal views of the mid cervical region; (c) axial view of the lower cervical region. (1) Sternomastoid. (2) Omohyoid. (3) Sternohyoid. (4) Internal jugular vein. (5) Common carotid artery. (6) Scalenus anterior. (7) Thyroid. (8) Sternothyroid. (9) Inferior thyroid artery. (10) Oesophagus.

as when examining the deep venous system of the leg, repeatedly compress the IJV (i.e. bounce the probe). This does two things: it easily identifies the compressible IJV and 'fixes' the IJV in the centre of the probe and subsequent field of view. When the mid and lower cervical regions are scanned, the oesophagus may be identified medial to the CCA and at times it is situated quite lateral to the trachea. It is more commonly seen on the left. Ask the patient to swallow to permit easy clarification.

Lower cervical region (see Figure 1.11c)

The point at which the omohyoid crosses the carotid artery marks the boundary of the lower cervical region.

Continue to scan inferiorly in the transverse plane, using the great vessels as key localising structures, to reach the junction of the subclavian and CCA. This marks the root of the neck; the origin of the subclavian artery can be seen by angling the probe inferiorly behind the medial head of the clavicle.

The key structure in the root of the neck is the scalenus anterior muscle. This muscle runs inferiorly from the transverse processes of the cervical spine, passing posterior to the IJV to dip behind the medial clavicle to attach to the first rib. Scanning the IJV transversely and then in the sagittal plane more inferiorly, it is possible to identify the scalenus anterior muscle posterior to the IJV running from 12 o'clock to 7 o'clock (on the patient's right). This muscle lies between the second

part of the subclavian artery posteriorly and the subclavian vein anteriorly.

The root of the neck is a difficult area to assess with ultrasound. The anatomy is more easily appreciated once the scalenus anterior and the subclavian artery are identified (Figure 1.12). By angling inferiorly one can identify reverberation artefact from the apex of the lung inferior to the subclavian artery (Figure 1.13d). The ideal combination is a patient with a relatively thin neck and a small footprint probe – a situation that is not always encountered.

Posterior triangle region (Figure 1.13)

Having reached the clavicle, one now heads northwards again to assess the posterior triangle region. Beginners in head and neck ultrasound are often daunted in their attempts at assessing the posterior triangle by the large number of muscles that instantly fill the screen. Where does one start?

Remember that the posterior triangle is a very superficial region of the neck, bordered anteriorly by the sternomastoid and posteriorly by the trapezius muscle. The floor is formed by muscles running obliquely: these are (from anterior to posterior) the scalene, levator scapulae and splenius capitis muscles. Covering the muscular floor is a carpet of cervical fascia. The contents of the posterior triangle which lie superficial to the fascial carpet are few: spinal accessory nerve (XI), spinal accessory lymph node chain, pre-axillary

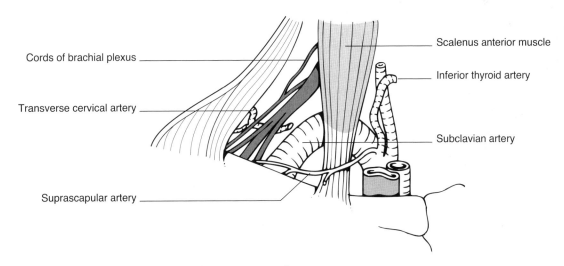

Cords of brachial plexus

Transverse cervical artery

Suprascapular artery

Scalenus anterior muscle

Inferior thyroid artery

Subclavian artery

Figure 1.12 – The key relationships of the scalenus anterior muscle.

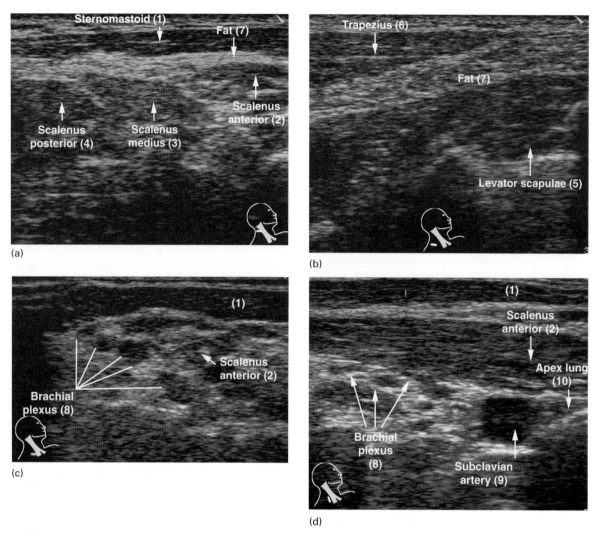

Figure 1.13 – (a, b) Axial views of the posterior triangle region; (c) axial view of the supraclavicular region; (d) sagittal view of the supraclavicular region. (1) Sternomastoid. (2) Scalenus anterior. (3) Scalenus medius. (4) Scalenus posterior. (5) Levator scapulae. (6) Trapezius. (7) Fat. (8) Brachial plexus. (9) Subclavian artery. (10) Apex lung.

brachial plexus, dorsal scapular nerve and fat. More inferiorly the transverse cervical artery and vein, arising from the thyrocervical trunk and IJV respectively, can be found coursing parallel to the clavicle.

Assessment is easy if it is remembered that the posterior triangle is a fat-filled superficial structure. The plane between the superficial sternomastoid and trapezius muscles and the deeper muscles of the posterior triangle floor is identified, and scanning is undertaken in a transverse plane from mastoid tip, i.e. sternomastoid origin, to mid/lateral clavicle. Remember that the spinal accessory nerve (and the accompanying lymph

node chain) runs from a point halfway between the mastoid process and angle of mandible to the outer third of the clavicle; maintaining the probe in that line will ensure that the territory of the spinal accessory chain is covered. On transverse scans, the tips of the transverse processes of the vertebrae may be seen as echogenic structures with posterior acoustic shadowing. Do not mistake these for calcified lymph nodes.

Supraclavicular region (see Figure 1.13c, d)

Once the probe has passed down along the line of the posterior triangle and come to rest at the lateral clavicle, the next area to examine is the supraclavicular region. The clavicle forms a convenient inferior border and it is logical to sweep medially with the probe held in a sagittal plane. The subclavian vein, situated superior and posterior to the clavicle, is a good landmark although it is not consistently seen.

The three major muscles to identify are the trapezius, omohyoid and sternomastoid. The distal trapezius is attached to the lateral clavicle; its anterior free border is easily recognised. The inferior belly of omohyoid is usually apparent due to its oblique plane. Just superior to the inferior belly of omohyoid are the transverse cervical artery and vein.

Moving medially, it is possible to identify the brachial plexus[8] with ultrasound (Figure 1.13c, d). Note the scalenus anterior muscle in the transverse plane, behind the IJV. Scanning inferiorly, rounded hypo-echoic structures will be seen emerging from behind the lateral border of scalenus anterior and passing laterally, just superior to the third portion of the subclavian artery. These represent the trunks of the brachial plexus.

Once the sternomastoid has been reached the examination of the supraclavicular region is complete.

Midline (Figure 1.14)

Most operators are comfortable with imaging of the thyroid. However, most fail to examine systematically the midline structures of the neck. If a comprehensive examination of the neck is to be achieved, it is important to examine the midline from mandible to sternum. The anatomy of the thyroid and larynx are dealt with in detail in Chapters 3 and 6, however a couple of areas which tend to be neglected by sonographers and radiologists are highlighted here.

Above the hyoid bone the anatomy is easy. The submental triangle is readily defined and the anatomy has been discussed earlier.

The larynx is an unfamiliar structure to image with US, but the operator should be able to ascertain some recognisable landmarks — these are the epiglottis and pre-epiglottic space, which are seen in sagittal sections. The cords, both false and true, can be identified in axial and parasagittal sections. The anatomy of the thyroid and parathyroids is discussed in Chapter 3.

The cricoid cartilage is a good landmark in the midline; it tends to lie just above the isthmus of the thyroid. It is a broad cartilaginous structure and can be identified in sagittal section in contrast to the finer cartilaginous tracheal rings that are seen more inferiorly. One should be able to identify these landmarks.

Ultrasound can be used to identify the trachea and its cartilaginous rings, allowing US-guided punctures of the trachea to be performed to facilitate percutaneous tracheostomy.[9,10] The optimal site is between the first and second tracheal rings. Percutaneous tracheostomy can be hazardous in an oedematous or obese neck. Ultrasound can identify the trachea and its rings (Figure 1.14) whilst also identifying other potential hazards such as a large thyroid isthmus or venous anomalies.

The strap muscles form a thin anterior covering of the midline structures and it is convenient to group these muscles together as 'strap muscles'. However a more detailed knowledge of the anatomy is required when trying to identify the exact location of thyroglossal duct cysts, anterior cervical chain nodes, etc. (Figure 1.15).

Now that the reader is familiar with a systematic approach to examining the neck, recognition of a series of landmarks should be possible. If this basic approach is used and modified according to the needs of the investigation, the beginner should be able to approach ultrasound scanning of the neck with a degree of confidence.

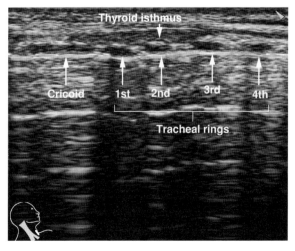

Figure 1.14 – The midline region.

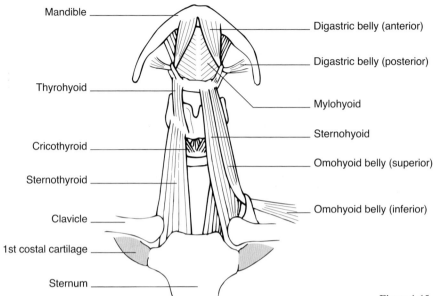

Mandible

Thyrohyoid

Cricothyroid

Sternothyroid

Clavicle

1st costal cartilage

Sternum

Digastric belly (anterior)

Digastric belly (posterior)

Mylohyoid

Sternohyoid

Omohyoid belly (superior)

Omohyoid belly (inferior)

Figure 1.15 – The strap muscles of the neck.

References

1. American Joint Committee on Cancer. *AJCC Cancer Staging Manual/American Joint Committee on Cancer,* 5th edn. New York: Lippincott-Raven, 1997.

2. Agur AMR. *Grant's Atlas of Anatomy,* 9th edn. Baltimore: Williams & Wilkins, 1991.

3. Harnsberger HR. *Handbook Of Head And Neck Imaging,* 2nd edn. Chicago: Mosby-Year Book, 1995.

4. Babbel RW, Harnsberger HR. The parapharyngeal space: The key to unlocking the suprahyoid neck. *Semin Ultrasound CT MR* 1990; **11:** 444–459.

5. Harnsberger HR, Osborn AG. Differential diagnosis of head and neck lesions based on their space of origin. 1: The suprahyoid part of the neck. *Ann J Roentgenol* 1991; **157:** 147–154.

6. Smoker WRK, Harnsberger HR. Differential diagnosis of head and neck lesions based on their space of origin. 2: The infrahyoid portion of the neck. *Ann J Roentgenol* 1991; **157:** 155–159.

7. Rhys R, Evans RM. Sonography of the submandibular duct. *Eur J Ultrasound* 1998; **8 (3):** S16. (Abst.)

8. Yang WT, Chui PT, Metreweli C. Anatomy of the normal brachial plexus revealed by sonography and the role of sonographic guidance in anaesthesia of the brachial plexus. *AJR* 1998; **171 (6):** 1631–1636.

9. Bertram S, Emshoff R, Norer B. Ultrasonographic anatomy of the anterior neck: Implications for tracheostomy. *J Oral Maxillofac Surg* 1995; **53:** 1420–1424.

10. Muhammad JK, Patton DW, Evans RM, Major E. Percutaneous dilatational tracheostomy (PDT) under ultrasound guidance. *Br J Oral Maxillofac Surg* 1999; **37:** 309–311.

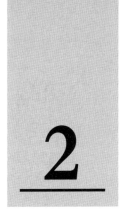

2

SALIVARY GLANDS

MJ Bradley

This chapter describes the normal salivary gland anatomy, highlighting the ultrasound features and landmarks. Patient preparation and techniques are outlined to avoid pitfalls in diagnosis.

The majority of cases present to the clinician and sonologist as a facial or neck lump, and this chapter outlines a diagnostic approach to the problem. The efficacy of ultrasound is described together with its interaction with other imaging modalities, mainly sialography, CT and MRI.[1]

> ### Contents Parotid space
> - parotid gland
> - facial nerve
> - retromandibular vein
> - external carotid artery
> - lymph nodes.

Normal anatomy

Parotid space

The parotid gland is a major paired gland for saliva production in the mouth. The gland lies in the parotid space, which is the most lateral space in the nasopharyngeal area. It extends from the external auditory canal superiorly to the level of the angle of the mandible inferiorly. The masticator, parapharyngeal and carotid spaces border the parotid space on its medial aspect from anterior to posterior. The posterior belly of the digastric muscle divides the carotid space from the parotid space. It is thus important to consider pathologies arising from these spaces when examining the 'parotid mass'.

FACIAL NERVE

The facial nerve creates an artificial plane to divide the gland into superficial and deep lobes. Accurate localisation of the mass is important in defining surgical approach both for adequate resection and in the preservation of the facial nerve.

Ultrasound is not yet able to identify definitively the facial nerve. However, with new generation equipment this may become a realistic prospect. MRI has attained limited views of the main facial nerve trunk but this is often mistaken for salivary ducts.[2,3]

The facial nerve runs antero-inferiorly and obliquely from the styloid foramen superiorly through the parotid gland. It lies superficial to the vascular plane, therefore the vascular plane is important in guiding the sonologist to the position of the facial nerve.

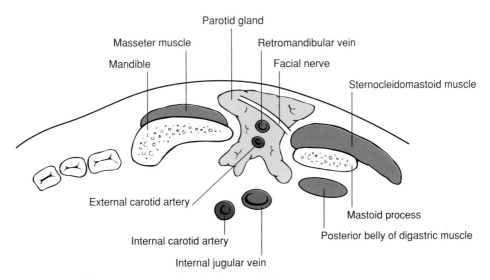

Figure 2.1 – Line drawing of a transverse section through the parotid gland.

VESSELS

The two main vessels run medial and parallel to the facial nerve with the external carotid artery being the most medial of the three structures (the retromandibular vein is sandwiched in the middle). These vessels are thus important landmarks for the plane of the facial nerve and in division of the superficial and deep lobes.[4] The vascular plane runs from supero-posteriorly to the inferior lateral pole.

LYMPH NODES

The parotid space contains multiple normal lymph nodes both within the parotid gland and outside the gland. These drain sites from the scalp, external auditory canal as well as deep facial spaces. The intraparotid nodes lie mainly in the superficial lobe but deep lobe nodes may also be seen. They are identified as round/oval hypo-echoic lesions, generally less than 5 mm in diameter and are usually well defined. An echogenic hilus differentiates the node from other parotid masses (Figure 2.2).

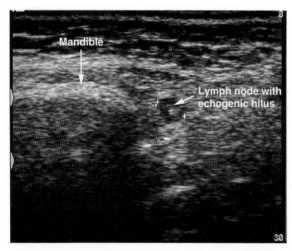

Figure 2.2 – Axial ultrasound image showing intraparotid node. Note (1) central echogenic hilus (arrowed) and (2) mandible (arrowed).

STENSEN'S DUCT

The intraglandular ducts drain into a main single duct which emerges from the anterior aspect of the gland to run over the superficial aspect of the masseter muscle. The main duct is visible as a fine echogenic line within the superficial lobe. At its anterior border, the duct then turns medially through the buccinator to enter the cheek mucosa at the level of the upper second molar.

> ## ULTRASOUND ANATOMY OF THE PAROTID SPACE
>
> 1 Homogeneous, hyperechoic gland.
> 2 Stensen's duct – bright parallel echogenic lines, no more than 3 mm in diameter. Normally not seen beyond the parenchyma.
> 3 Intraglandular ducts – short discrete hyperechoic thin lines within the gland parenchyma.
> 4 Retromandibular vein – running obliquely through the gland as a well-defined hypoechoic tube. Landmark for facial nerve.
> 5 External carotid artery is deep and parallel to the vein.
> 6 Posterior belly of digastric – demarcates carotid space boundary.
> 7 Intraparotid lymph nodes – round/oval, < 5 mm diameter, echogenic hilus. Commonly lie in superficial lobe but may also be seen in the deep lobe.

Submandibular space (Figure 2.3)

The oral cavity contains two major spaces: the sublingual space and the submandibular space. The mylohyoid muscle divides the two spaces; the submandibular space is located inferolateral to the mylohyoid muscle whilst the sublingual space lies superomedially. The submandibular gland has superficial and deep lobes but imaging is not normally required to differentiate between them as the surgical options are invariably the same for any submandibular mass.

Contents:

Submandibular space:

- anterior belly of digastric muscle
- superficial lobe submandibular gland
- lymph nodes (submandibular and submental)
- facial artery and vein
- inferior loop of XII nerve
- fat.

Sublingual space:

- anterior hyoglossus muscle
- deep lobe of submandibular gland
- sublingual gland and ducts

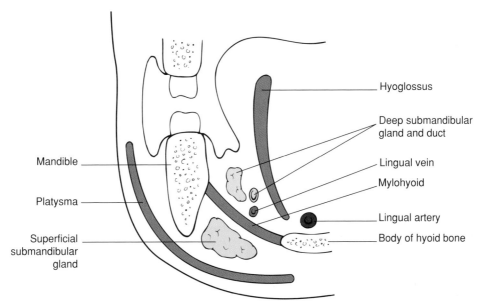

Figure 2.3 – Line drawing of a coronal section through the submandibular gland. The mylohyoid defines the floor of the mouth and demarcates the submandibular space. The hyoglossus is the key for identifying the submandibular duct. The anterior belly of the digastric demarcates the submental space. The anterior facial vein lies posterior to the submandibular gland and is useful for differentiating between parotid and submandibular origin of a mass.

- submandibular duct (Wharton's)
- lingual artery and vein
- lingual nerve
- cranial nerves IX and XII.

Salivary gland technique

1 The scan plane is mainly transverse (axial) with oblique or longitudinal adjustments to confirm vessels and to help localise lesions.

2 Have the patient sit or recline with the neck extended. The patient's head should be turned contralaterally for best access. A water bath or stand-off medium is not usually necessary except for postoperative or post-radiotherapy patients. Extremely superficial lesions are sometimes visualised better with a stand-off medium.

3 Always scan both sides for symmetry and to exclude further clinically non-palpable lesions as there is a risk of bilateral disease.

4 Scan all nodal territories.

ULTRASOUND ANATOMY OF THE SUB-MANDIBULAR & SUBLINGUAL SPACES

1 Homogeneous hyperechogenicity similar to the parotid glands. The sublingual glands demonstrate similar echogenicity to the other salivary glands.

2 Wharton's duct – this is seen when it is abnormally dilated (Figure 2.4) but it may occasionally be seen in normal cases. The duct extends from the gland hilus medially to curve around the mylohyoid muscle, appearing lateral to the hyoglossus muscle. It then advances medially to the papilla in the floor of the mouth.

3 The intraglandular ducts appear as in the parotid, i.e. short, defined hyperechoic lines.

4 The anterior division of the retromandibular vein is sandwiched between the posterior pole of the submandibular gland and the antero-inferior margin of the parotid gland. This landmark may be important when it is displaced by a large mass, giving a further indication as to the origin of the lesion, i.e. parotid or submandibular.

5 The sublingual glands are easily visualised submentally deep to the mylohyoid and lateral to the geniohyoid/genioglossus.

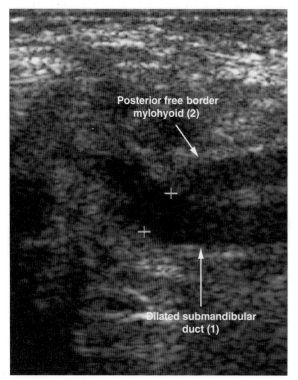

Figure 2.4 – Transverse image. (1) Dilated submandibular duct (arrowed) swerving around (2) posterior border of mylohyoid (arrowed).

5 Start the scan with known ultrasound landmarks then work towards the underlying lesion.

Pitfalls of technique

- It can be difficult to scan the entire deep lobe of the parotid because of the bony anatomy. Rotate or angle the probe, or move the patient's neck to obtain best access.

- Large masses may reduce confidence of complete visualisation and origin. If the margins of the mass cannot be defined, proceed to CT or MRI.

- When the patient is swallowing, trapped bubbles in the floor of the mouth may simulate submandibular calculi.

- The greater cornu of the hyoid may be mistaken for calcification/calculi if anatomical landmarks are not followed.

Calculi and acute inflammatory disease

Sialolithiasis (Figures 2.4–2.7)

Submandibular calculi are more common than parotid calculi. The greater number (80%) of calculi that occur in the submandibular gland are attributed to the greater mucous content of the submandibular saliva,[5] parotid saliva tending to be more aqueous. 90% of sub-mandibular calculi are radio-opaque, whereas only 10% of parotid stones are radio-opaque. The majority of patients present with a solitary calculus; however, multiple calculi are found in 3% of patients.

High sensitivity (94%), specificity (100%) and accuracy (96%) are claimed for the detection of calculi by ultra-sound.[6] Such accuracy can only stem from meticulous technique. Intraglandular calculi are easier to detect than ductal stones but, as discussed previously, it is

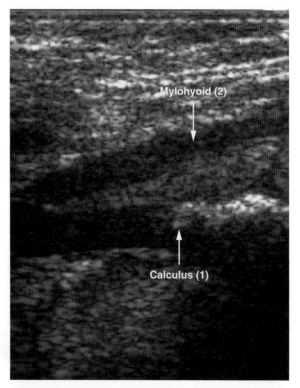

Figure 2.5 – Transverse image. (1) Calculus demonstrated within distal duct (arrow), with proximal sludge. (2) Mylohyoid (arrowed).

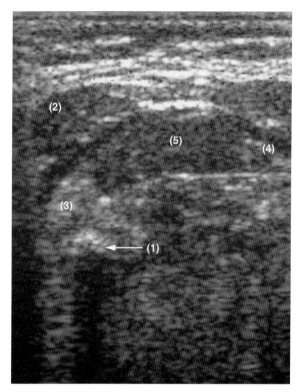

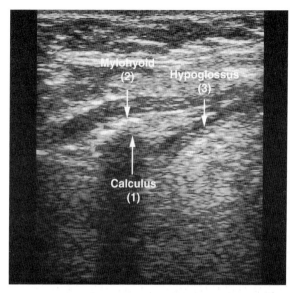

Figure 2.7 – Coronal oblique image showing (1) calculus (arrowed) in proximal duct sandwiched between (2) mylohyoid (arrow) and (3) hyoglossus (arrow) muscles.

Figure 2.6 – Coronal section. (1) Stone demonstrated in distal duct (arrowed). Note relationship to (2) anterior belly digastric and (3) echogenic sublingual gland (4) mylohyoid and (5) genio-hyoid also demonstrated.

important to remember the key anatomy when look-ing for ductal calculi.

In the parotid gland the main duct is easily identified as parallel echogenic lines. Ductal stones can be identified if one remembers that the main duct continues approximately one finger breadth below the zygomatic arch until it pierces the buccinator muscle, and scan-ning should take place in this plane.

The plane of the submandibular duct is more difficult to locate: the key to identifying the proximal duct is the hyoglossus muscle. Scan in the coronal plane and identify the mylohyoid muscle and hyoglossus muscle more medially; the proximal duct will be sandwiched between the two, together with the lingual vein. Identify the vein with colour flow then gently rotate the probe while keeping the duct central until a trans-verse plane is reached with the duct identified lateral to hyoglossus. The distal duct is not usually identified

unless it is dilated. It opens into the floor of the mouth approximately one centimetre behind the attachment of the anterior belly of digastric muscle to the mandible. A coronal scan looking just posterior to the anterior belly of digastric muscle should identify any distal calculi, surrounded by the hyperechoic lingual gland.

Ultrasound may demonstrate sialectasis; a hypoechoic parenchyma with prominent intraglandular ducts is typical.[7] Frank duct dilatation can be seen, usually when the duct calculus is also identified.[8] The compli-cations of calculi, namely sialocele and abscess, may also be identified with ultrasound.[9] Duct strictures are best diagnosed at sialography.

Ultrasound can in many instances give the surgeon all the information required, obviating the need for sialography. Intraglandular or proximal duct stones are dealt with via a cervical approach (Figure 2.8), whereas an intra-oral approach will be used if stones are identified in the distal submandibular or parotid duct. Duct calculi may be removed radiologically using balloons or baskets, and lithotripsy is also being used.[10]

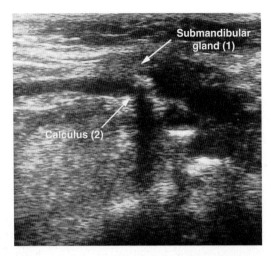

Figure 2.8 – Chronic sialadenitis of (1) submandibular gland (arrowed) with (2) calculus demonstrated in proximal duct (arrow).

SIALOLITHIASIS
Parenchymal/duct calculi – surgery or radiologically guided balloon/basket extraction
Duct dilatation – sialography to identify small duct stones or duct stricture
Sialectasis – sialography if obstructive history
Abscess/infection – ultrasound-guided aspiration of pus

Hypertrophy

Ultrasound shows bilateral salivary gland enlargement with a normal echogenicity. Sometimes the glands are hyperechoic due to fatty infiltration. This may be seen in obesity, alcoholism, diabetes or uraemia. Fatty infiltration can be seen in normal adults; having an ethnic bias, and is commonly seen in North Africans. Various dietary and metabolic disorders as well as drugs can cause parotid enlargement. A prominent accessory lobe of the parotid may be seen as a normal variant.

Acute inflammation

The parotid is the salivary gland most commonly affected by acute suppurative sialadenitis; the likely causes are stone, stricture or dehydration. The organism is usually *Staphylococcus aureus*, but *Strep. pneumoniae*, *E. coli* and *Haemophilus influenzae* have also been isolated. Tuberculosis may cause granulomatous inflammatory disease, as may actinomycosis, syphilis, blastomycosis and histoplasmosis; however, these conditions are rare.[11]

The acutely inflamed salivary gland shows enlargement and hypo-echogenicity on ultrasound scanning. The parenchyma may have a heterogeneous pattern attributable to the presence of micro-abscesses or localised duct dilatation/retention cysts. Progression to an abscess results in an ill-defined hypo-echogenicity within the gland, sometimes with frank fluid content. There may be hyperechoic foci due to microbubbles of gas within the abscess. Prior to liquefaction, the abscess will appear as an ill-defined hypo-echoic inflammatory mass. The bright intraglandular ducts are clearly seen inside the lesion, indicating that the lesion is ill defined and permeates through the gland rather than causing duct displacement as per tumour. Painful parotid or neck nodes are often present and it is possible that these may also liquefy and produce further abscesses. Ultrasound-guided aspiration allows appropriate antibiotic therapy to be introduced; in the case of unilocular abscesses it may avoid the need for surgery.

ULTRASOUND APPEARANCES IN ACUTE INFLAMMATION
Sialadenitis – heterogeneous, hypo-echoic gland, micro-abscesses
Inflammatory mass – hypo-echoic, ill-defined gland, ducts within lesion
Abscess – frank fluid, gas microbubbles

Viral infections

Viruses, in particular the mumps virus, are the most frequent causes of salivary gland swelling. Viral infection is usually a clinical diagnosis, not requiring any imaging. Ultrasound shows unilateral or bilateral gland enlargement, often hypo-echoic in texture. Cervical nodes are common. Viral infections may cause a chronic sialadenitis which can cause recurrent parotitis (Figure 2.9).[12] The main reason for the ultrasound scan is to exclude an abscess in what may be a difficult clinical assessment (Figure 2.10).

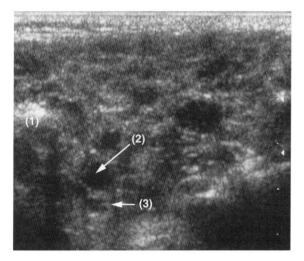

Figure 2.9 – Axial section of the parotid showing multiple rounded hypo-echoic areas within a heterogeneous parenchyma. Note (1) mandible, (2) retromandibular vein (arrowed), (3) external carotid artery (arrowed). Diagnosis: Juvenile chronic sialadenitis.

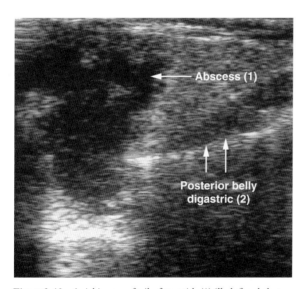

Figure 2.10 – Axial image of tail of parotid: (1) ill-defined abscess with internal debris (arrowed). Aspiration yielded pus. Double arrow – (2) posterior belly digastric.

Chronic inflammatory conditions

Sjögren's syndrome (Figures 2.11, 2.12)

Sjögren's syndrome is a common auto-immune condition seen almost exclusively in women. The patients are usually middle-aged females who present with dry eyes and mouth.

In the early stages the salivary glands may be normal or show diffuse enlargement with normal echogenicity. The late features are virtually diagnostic: a heterogeneous echo texture with multiple round hypo-echoic

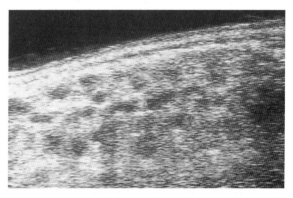

Figure 2.11 – Sjögren's disease of superficial parotid. Rounded hypo-echoic areas with relatively normal background parenchyma.

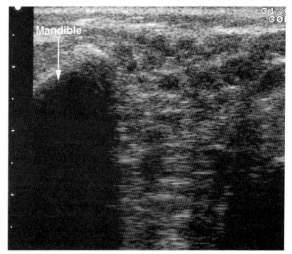

Figure 2.12 – Sjögren's disease. Axial section of parotid showing multiple rounded hypo-echoic areas distributed throughout the gland. Note similar appearances to sialadenitis. (Figure 2.9). Mandible (arrowed).

areas within the parenchyma, sometimes also containing frank cystic changes.[13] In longstanding disease there is atrophy of the glands, which then appear as small and hypo-echoic.[14,15] Increased perfusion as assessed by colour Doppler may reflect the severity of the morphological changes.[16]

The role of ultrasound in Sjögren's disease is two-fold: (a) to confirm or exclude salivary gland involvement; (b) to look for lymphomatous change, as there is an association of lymphoma with Sjögren's syndrome.

Sialography may show punctate parenchymal opacification and intravasation due to disorganised duct epithelium. Scintigraphy can be helpful for monitoring the response to therapy. However, these modalities probably have little extra to offer in making the diagnosis.[17]

Sarcoidosis

Sarcoidosis is a rare clinical finding in the salivary gland (6%) but is histologically present in 33% of patients with sarcoidosis. It may present as a lump, with or without local pain. Ultrasound is non-specific but may show diffuse hypo-echogenicity in a normal sized or enlarged gland. The submandibular gland is the favoured site. It is likely that the gland will be excised for a histological diagnosis unless, as in some instances, the diagnosis has already been established by other means, i.e. core biopsy. Heerfordt's syndrome is an unusual form of sarcoidosis consisting of uveiitis, parotid swelling and facial paralysis.

Radiotherapy

Radiotherapy of the neck may result in localised pain or swelling in the salivary glands. This is more common in the submandibular gland. In the acute phase the gland is enlarged and hypo-echoic whereas chronic change results in a small atrophied, hypo-echoic gland.

Trauma

Trauma to the salivary glands usually involves the parotid gland. The clinically important anatomical structures in this situation are the external carotid artery, the facial nerve and Stensen's duct. CT is probably the optimal initial imaging modality, but ultrasound may help to assess a sialocele or haematoma. Sialography may best image the Stensen's duct injury, however ultrasound can demonstrate transection of the duct (Figure 2.13) and help in the assessment of fistulae.

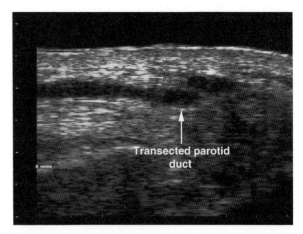

Figure 2.13 – Axial image showing transected distal parotid duct (arrowed). Injury sustained following an assault with a broken glass.

Salivary gland tumours

The patient's symptoms usually relate to a palpable lump or pain. Up to 20% of clinically diagnosed salivary gland masses are found to be due to lesions outside the salivary gland by ultrasound (Figure 2.14).[18] The incidence of salivary gland tumours is less than 3 per 10^5 head of population, although there are recognised geographic variations. Salivary gland tumours are more commonly seen in the parotid; 85–90% of these are benign. The clinical parameters for malignancy are rapidly growing lesions, nodal enlargement and facial nerve paralysis. However, because submandibular masses have a greater propensity for malignancy (33%), the sonologist should have a lower threshold of suspicion for malignant tumours in the submandibular or sublingual spaces.

The sonologist should beware of a large tumour or one arising from the deep lobe (less than 10% of cases).[19] It is not always easy to accurately assess the extent of the lesion in these circumstances, and CT or MRI will be required. Occasionally a deep space mass, (parapharyngeal, carotid or masticator space) may displace or invade the parotid and simulate a parotid mass on clinical examination. The sonologist needs to assess whether the boundaries of the mass can be defined or whether only the 'tip of the iceberg' is being imaged. Deep lobe masses appear medial to the mandible and vascular plane and cause predominantly lateral duct displacement. Ultrasound is as effective as other modalities in the role of tumour localisation.[20]

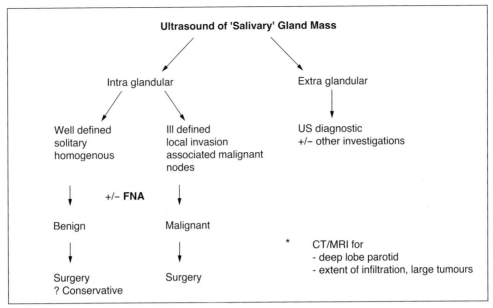

Figure 2.14 – Ultrasound of 'salivary gland' mass.

The origin of the mass is important not only in the differential diagnosis but also in guiding the surgical approach to the patient – a transparotid approach with identification of the facial nerve, or a peri-oral or submandibular incision for an extraparotid mass.

The ultrasound distinction of benign and malignant lesions is not precise but suspicion should be aroused when the lesion is ill defined or locally invading, when it is in the deep lobe, and when neck nodes are present. Ultrasound is able to evaluate a benign lesion in over 80% of cases.[21] Colour Doppler may also aid in the assessment of malignancy; the lesion with a disorganised colour Doppler pattern and RI >0.8, PI >2 is more likely to be malignant. Prediction of malignancy may affect the surgical approach, and the diagnosis may be enhanced by fine-needle aspiration (FNA).[22]

SALIVARY GLAND TUMOURS

Intraparotid or extraparotid?
Well defined or ill defined?
Local invasion?
Superficial or deep lobe?
Single or multiple?
Complete boundaries on ultrasound?
Need for other imaging?
Facial nerve?
Nodes?

Benign tumours

PLEOMORPHIC ADENOMA

Pleomorphic adenoma is the most common of the parotid tumours (60–80%). Histology reveals a mixture of epithelial and myo-epithelial cells, hence its common name of 'benign mixed tumour'. The patient is typically more than 40 years old and complains of a slowly growing mass. It is more common in women and is ten times more frequent in the parotid than in the submandibular gland. 90% of parotid pleomorphic adenomas arise in the superficial lobe and are frequently assessed adequately by ultrasound alone.

It is claimed that in up to 25% of pleomorphic adenomas small satellite foci can be demonstrated separate from the main mass.[23] This has fuelled debate over a multicentric origin of this disease.

Pleomorphic adenoma is usually treated by a superficial parotid lobectomy but there is a propensity for recurrence. In some instances this may occur because the multicentric nature of the tumour has not been identified, with the result that it is incompletely resected.

The ultrasound appearance is that of a hypo-echoic solid mass which is round or oval and well defined with a lobulated or bosselated surface. Typically the pleomorphic adenoma is less than 3 cm in diameter, hypo-echoic, homogeneous, well defined and often displays 'through' transmission (Figures 2.15, 2.16).

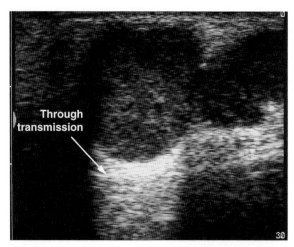

Figure 2.15 – Typical 'through' transmission (arrowed) demonstrated in multicentric pleomorphic adenomata within the parotid.

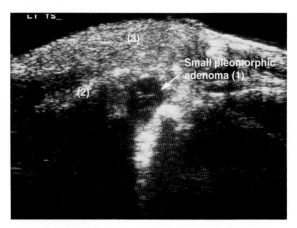

Figure 2.16 – Axial image using 5 MHz probe showing (1) small pleomorphic adenoma in deep lobe (arrowed). Note (2) mandible, (3) superficial lobe parotid.

This should not lead to it being confused with a cyst – colour Doppler may demonstrate intratumour flow, or FNA can confirm its non-cystic nature. The 'through' transmission is probably caused by an artefact – hyperechoic parenchyma surrounding a markedly hypo-echoic mass. Also, the mass effect of the lesion leading to duct displacement and crowding may make the deep wall of the lesion echogenically brighter. Malignancy should be considered when the lesion is poorly defined or there is frank local invasion. Lack of homogeneity should also be regarded as suspi-

cious. The pleomorphic adenoma is generally regarded as a benign lesion; some suggest that it has malignant potential, but this is contentious.

Large tumours (> 3 cm) are more prone to cystic or haemorrhagic degeneration, which may cause reduced homogeneity on ultrasound. Calcification may also occur in longstanding tumour.

Neck nodes are not normally associated with pleomorphic adenoma.

PLEOMORPHIC ADENOMA
Female patient > 40 years
Homogeneous, hypo-echoic
Well-defined, round, lobulated
'Through' transmission
Peripheral colour flow Doppler pattern
Multicentric

The colour Doppler pattern of the pleomorphic adenoma is variable but commonly shows increased peripheral vessels, mainly venous.[24] This pattern may be seen with malignancy and so cannot be regarded as diagnostic. However RI < 0.8 and PI < 2.0 favour a benign lesion.[25]

WARTHIN'S TUMOUR (ADENOLYMPHOMA)

This tumour accounts for 6–10% of parotid tumours. It typically presents in the elderly male (> 50 years) as a lump in the parotid tail. It is rarely seen in the submandibular gland. The tumour arises from heterotopic salivary gland tissue in parotid lymph nodes. It has an excellent prognosis and does not tend to recur if resected. Indeed many 'Warthin's tumours' may undergo surveillance without resort to surgery; FNA is thus particularly helpful if surgery is contraindicated (Figure 2.17). Less than 15% are bilateral.

On ultrasound, a Warthin's tumour is typically well circumscribed and usually less than 3 cm in diameter. It may show internal heterogeneity of solid and cystic areas. Indeed, a lesion that appears well defined and shows a multiseptated cystic architecture may be diagnosed as a Warthin's tumour with a high degree of specificity. This 'classical' appearance, however, is unusual.[26] Warthin's tumour may also appear anechoic with through transmission. It is often mistaken ultrasonically for a pleomorphic adenoma. Colour flow

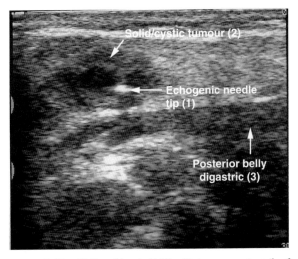

Figure 2.17 – FNA of 'typical' Warthin's tumour in tail of parotid. Note (1) echogenic needle tip, (2) solid/cystic tumour, (3) posterior belly digastric.

Doppler may show vessels in a hilar distribution with branches in the septa of the structure.[25]

WARTHIN'S TUMOUR
Male > 50 years
Hypo- or anechoic, well defined
'Through' transmission
Multiseptated cystic architecture
Bilateral
Apex/tail of superficial lobe

ONCOCYTOMA

This uncommon tumour appears exclusively in the older adult (> 50 years). It is a solid tumour composed of oncocytes (large cells with granular eosinophilic cytoplasm) and is found in the parotid. There are no specific ultrasound features; it is similar in appearance to the other benign lesions.

OTHER BENIGN TUMOURS

These lesions arise within the glandular spaces from non-parenchymatous elements. They include lipomas and vascular tumours. The lipoma is well defined and hyperechoic. Its compressible nature and bright streaks

parallel to the skin surface are useful diagnostic features. CT and MRI are diagnostic as they demonstrate characteristic fatty attenuation or signal.

Haemangiomas are more frequently seen in children or young adults. They may also be compressible and may give a bluish skin discolouration. They may change in size with posture or crying. The ultrasound shows an inhomogeneous lesion which is usually poorly defined.[27] Vascular spaces or associated abnormally large vessels may occasionally be recognised. Focal calcification (phleboliths) may be identified in some instances. Colour Doppler is generally unhelpful as the internal flow is typically sluggish and thus it is difficult to demonstrate such low flow velocities. Colour 'fill in' may be observed upon release of pressure after compression of the mass.

Red cell labelled scintigraphy is diagnostic if there is a clinical dilemma.[27]

Malignant salivary gland tumours

Malignant epithelial tumours of the salivary glands account for 17% of all epithelial tumours. The smaller salivary glands have greater malignant potential, a tumour in the sublingual or submandibular gland being more likely to be malignant than a tumour in the parotid.

Ultrasound alone may predict malignancy in 80–89% of cases.[28] The ultrasound features are similar for all malignant lesions and it is not possible to differentiate between the histological types.

MUCO-EPIDERMOID CARCINOMA

Muco-epidermoid carcinoma accounts for 5–10% of all salivary gland tumours, the majority arising from the parotid (80%). It occurs at any age and there is no sex predominance. It is the most common malignant tumour of childhood.

Most of these tumours are slow growing and present as firm or hard lesions. There is a marked tendency for local invasion. Pain or itching in the facial nerve territory is indicative of a malignant parotid tumour.

Muco-epidermoid carcinoma arises from ductal epithelium. The histological grade relates to the clinical picture: a low-grade tumour may feel and look like a benign lesion. Similarly, low-grade lesions may appear well defined whilst those of high grade are poorly defined and may be frankly infiltrative (Figure 2.18). It is difficult to discriminate the benign or

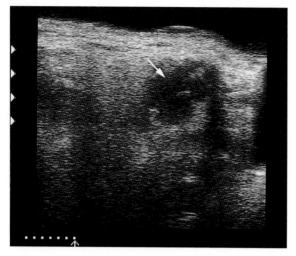

Figure 2.18 – Ill-defined heterogeneous tumour in superficial lobe of parotid (arrowed). Muco-epidermoid carcinoma.

malignant nature of a small encapsulated lesion using ultrasound, but larger tumours tend to have a more complex heterogeneous internal echopattern. This inhomogeneity reflects necrosis or haemorrhage within the tumour. Ultrasound also detects any nodal metastases in the neck. Colour Doppler is more likely to show pronounced vascularisation.[29]

CT or MRI may be needed to assess the presence of local spread, particularly to detect perineural extension along the facial nerve.

ADENOID CYSTIC CARCINOMA

Adenoid cystic carcinoma arises from peripheral ducts in the parotid gland; it accounts for 3% of parotid tumours and up to 17% of submandibular tumours. It tends to show infiltration (Figure 2.19) and is prone to perineural spread; even small peripheral tumours invade proximal nerve fibres. Ultrasound shows similar features to the muco-epidermoid carcinoma and CT or MRI may be required to assess local infiltration. Adenoid cystic carcinomas are more common in women over 40 years and appear as solitary round tumours accompanied by pain or facial nerve involvement.

ACINIC CELL CARCINOMA

Acinic cell carcinoma accounts for 2–4% of salivary gland malignancies. It arises from the terminal portion of the duct system and is likely to give rise to multiple lesions. Ultrasound may show intratumour cystic areas but otherwise the features are non-specific.

MALIGNANT TUMOURS
- Ill-defined/locally invasive
- Inhomogeneous and hypo-echoic
- Associated malignant nodes
- Disorganised colour flow, RI > 0.8, PI > 2

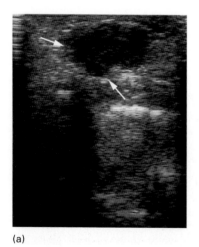

(a)

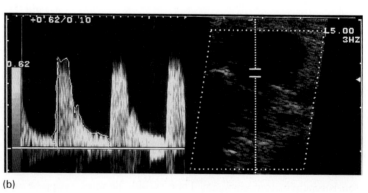

(b)

Figure 2.19 – Adenocarcinoma of parotid. Heterogeneous, hypo-echoic tumour with irregular margins (arrowed). Note high peak systolic velocity with a high resistance spectral trace.

METASTATIC TUMOUR

The parotid gland contains lymph nodes because of its embryologically late encapsulation. These nodes drain the lateral face and scalp and external auditory meatus which explains why squamous carcinoma and melanomas of the skin in these areas may metastasise to the parotid gland (Figure 2.20). They are often seen as small well-defined lesions and only their multiplicity and growth may give a clue to their true malignant nature. If there is no relevant history of a primary tumour to alert the clinician, then FNA/core biopsy may provide a histological diagnosis.

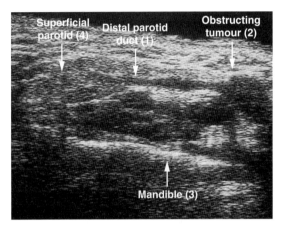

Figure 2.20 – Oblique image showing (1) dilated parotid duct due to (2) obstructing tumour (3) Mandible and (4) superficial parotid gland identified.

NON-HODGKIN'S LYMPHOMA

Non-Hodgkin's lymphoma usually involves the parotid nodes but may rarely give rise to extranodal disease in the salivary gland parenchyma. Multiple nodes are often also seen in all areas of the neck. Solitary nodes are unusual for lymphoma. Lymphomatous nodes are typically very hypo-echoic or anechoic and may show 'through' transmission. They are large and multiple.[30] Colour flow Doppler shows marked vascularity within these nodes.

Miscellaneous 'parotid' lesions

The sonologist not infrequently finds that the origin of the parotid mass is within the masseter muscle rather

than in the parotid gland. A history of recent dental treatment may alert one to the diagnosis of a masseter muscle abscess. Ultrasound shows a well-defined anechoic lesion in the masseter, with or without frank fluid collection (Figure 2.21). The diagnosis of abscess is achieved by the history of pain, dental sepsis or pus aspirated at FNA. FNA creates the opportunity for diagnosis of an abscess and identification of the organism as well as definitive drainage which may obviate the need for surgery.

Other focal masseter muscle lesions include tumour, which is usually metastatic. Breast or bronchial carcinoma and melanoma are the most common primaries. Frank bone destruction or periosteal reaction may be diagnostic for malignancy. Both can be detected with ultrasound, but radiography (namely an orthopantomogram) still has a significant role.

The most common tumour in the masseter muscle is the haemangioma. The ultrasound features are those of any peripheral haemangioma: hypo-echoic, ill-defined and compressible, with phleboliths. Vessels are sometimes seen but colour flow is often negative because of low flow velocities.

Unilateral masseter muscle hypertrophy may be easily diagnosed on ultrasound. The muscle shows normal echogenicity but the belly is significantly thickened compared to the non-symptomatic side. Occasionally masseter muscle hypertrophy may be bilateral; this makes it harder to appreciate the thickening but the clinical presentation should alert to the diagnosis.

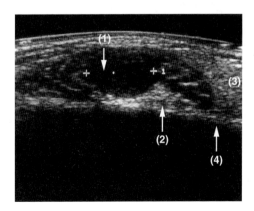

Figure 2.21 – (1) Masseter muscle abscess (arrowed). Note (2) masseter, (3) parotid, and (4) mandible.

> **MASSETER MUSCLE MASS**
> - Hypertrophy
> - Abscess
> - Tumour: primary – haemangioma; secondary – breast, bronchus, melanoma

Other mass lesions

Cystic masses of the salivary glands are rare.[31] The majority occur in the parotid gland (< 5% of all lesions). Congenital cysts arise from the first or second branchial groove and are most commonly seen in the infant. The other rare congenital cyst is the dermoid, consisting of keratinising squamous epithelium. Ultrasound shows an anechoic well-defined lesion. Acquired cysts may be seen in AIDS patients and mostly in children (benign lympho-epithelial cysts) as well as in conjunction with trauma, parotitis and calculi.[32,33] Some lympho-epithelial nodules in HIV-positive patients may demonstrate solid and cystic components resembling tumours.[34]

Mucus retention cysts with a true epithelial lining are rare but may arise with parotid duct obstruction. Mucoceles on the other hand are not true cysts and tend to occur in the sublingual gland (ranula).

References

1. Zhao Y, Zhang R. Differential diagnosis of parotid gland masses by grey scale real-time ultrasound. *Hua His I Ko Ta Hsueh Hsueh Pao* 1990; **21:** 92–95.

2. Tevesi LM, Kolin E, Lufkin RB, Hanafee WN. MR imaging of the intraparotid facial nerve: normal anatomy and pathology. *AJR* 1987; **148:** 995–1000.

3. Mandelblatt SM, Braun IF, Davis PC, Fry SM, Jacobs LH, Hoffman JC. Parotid masses: MR imaging. *Radiology* 1987; **163:** 411–414.

4. Laing MR, McKerrow WS. Intraparotid anatomy of the facial nerve and retromandibular vein. *Br J Surg* 1988; **75:** 310–312.

5. Rice DH. Advances in diagnosis and management of salivary gland diseases (Medical Progress). *West J Med* 1984; **140:** 238–249.

6. Gritzmann N. Sonography of the salivary glands. *AJR* 1989; **53:** 161–166.

7. Angelli G, Fana G, Macanini L, Lacaita MG, Laforgia A. Echography in the study of sialolithiasis. *Radiol Med Torino* 1990; **79:** 220–223.

8. Yoshimura Y, Inone Y, Odagana T. Sonographic evaluation of sialolithiasis. *J Oral Maxillofac Surg* 1989; **47:** 907–912.

9. Rubartelli L, Sponga T, Candiani F, Pittarello F, Andretta M. Infantile recurrent sialolectatic parotitis: the role of sonography and sialography in diagnosis and follow-up. *Br J Radiol* 1987; **60:** 1211–1214.

10. Iro H, Schneider T, Nitsche N, Waitz G, Marienhagen J, Ell C. Extra-corporeal shock wave lithotripsy of a salivary stone. *Dtsch Med Wochenschr* 1990; **115:** 12–14.

11. Epker BN. Obstructive and inflammatory diseases of the major salivary glands. *Oral Surg* 1972; **33 (1):** 2–27.

12. Nozaki H, Harasawa A, Hara H, Kohno A, Shigeta A. Ultrasonographic features of recurrent parotitis in childhood. *Pediatr Radiol* 1994; **24 (2):** 98–100.

13. Bradus RJ, Hybarjer P, Gooding GA. Parotid gland: US findings in Sjögren's syndrome. *Radiology* 1988; **169:** 749–751.

14. Corthours B, De Clerck LS, Francz L, De Schepper A, Vercruysse HA, Stevens WJ. Ultrasonography of the salivary glands in the evaluation of Sjögren's syndrome. Comparison with sialography. *J Belge Radiol* 1991; **74:** 189–192.

15. Kawamura H, Tanigudi N, Itoh K, Kano S. Salivary gland echography in patients with Sjögren's syndrome. *Arthritis Rheum* 1990; **33:** 505–510.

16. Steiner E, Graninger W, Hitzelhammer J, Lakits A, Petera P, Franz P, Gritzmann N. Colour coded duplex sonography of the parotid gland in Sjögren's syndrome (German). *Rofo Fortschr Geb Rontgenstr Neuen Bildgeb Verfahr* 1994; **160 (4):** 294–298.

17. Makula E, Pokorny G, Rajtar M, Kiss I, Kovacs A, Kovacs L. Parotid gland ultrasonography as a diagnostic tool in primary Sjögren's syndrome. *Br J Rheumatol* 1996; **35 (10):** 972–977.

18. Klein K, Turk R, Gritzmann N, Traxler M. The value of sonography in salivary gland tumours. *HNO* 1989; **37:** 71–75.

19. Da-Xi S, Ha Xiong S, Qiang Y. The diagnostic value of ultrasonography and salivography in salivary gland masses. *Dentomaxillofac Radiol* 1987; **16:** 37–45.

20. Bradley MJ, Ahuja A, Metreweli C. Sonic evaluation of the parotid ducts: its use in tumour localisation. *Br J Radiol* 1991; **64:** 1092–1095.

21. Bruneton JN, Mourou MY. Ultrasound in salivary gland disease. *ORL J Otorhinolaryngol Relat Spec* 1993; **55 (5):** 284–289.

22. Cardillo MR. Salivary gland masses: the diagnostic value of fine needle aspiration cytology. *Arch Anat Cytol Pathol* 1990; **38:** 26–32.

23. Bruneton JN, Normand R, Santini N, Balu-Maestro C. *Ultrasonography of the neck.* Berlin: Springer, 1987; ch 4, pp 66–79.

24. Martinoli C, Derchi LE, Solbiati L, Rizzatto G, Silvestri E, Giannoni M. Colour doppler sonography of salivary glands. *AJR* 1994; **163:** 933–941.

25. Bradley MJ. Colour flow doppler in the investigation of salivary gland tumours. *Abs/Eu J U/S* 1998; **7 Suppl 2:** S16.

26. Whyte AM, Byrne JV. A comparison of computed tomography and ultrasound in the assessment of parotid masses. *Clin Radiol* 1987; **38:** 339–343.

27. Bradley M, Stewart I, King W, Metreweli C. The role of ultrasound and ^{99}Tc RBC scintigraphy in the diagnosis of the salivary gland haemangioma. *Br Oral Maxillofac Surg* 1991; **29:** 164–165.

28. Wittich GR, Scheible WF, Haget PC. Ultrasonography of the salivary glands. *Radiol Clin North Am* 1985; **23**: 29–37.

29. Benzel W, Zenk J, Iro H. Colour Doppler ultrasound studies of parotid tumours (German). *HNO* 1995; **43 (1):** 25–30.

30. Bruneton JN, Caramella E, Roux P, Fenart D, Manzino JJ. Comparison of ultrasonographic and histological findings for multinodular lesions of the salivary glands. *Eur J Radiol* 1985; **5:** 295–296.

31. Work WP. Cysts and congenital lesions of the parotid gland. *Otolaryngol Clin North Am* 1977; **10:** 339.

32. Goddart D, Francois A, Ninare J, Vemylen C, Cornu G, Clapyyt P, Claus D. The parotid gland abnormality found in children seropositive for human immunodeficiency virus. *Paediatr Radiol* 1990; **20:** 355–357.

33. Shugar JM, Som PM, Jacobson AL, Ryan JR, Bernard PJ, Dickman SH. Multicentric parotid cysts and cervical adenopathy in AIDS patients. A newly recognized entity: CT and MR manifestations. *Laryngoscope* 1988; **98:** 772–775.

34. Martinoli C, Pretolesi F, Del Bono V, Derchi LE, Mecca D, Chiaramondia M. Benign lymphoepithelial parotid lesions in HIV-positive patients: spectrum of findings at gray-scale and doppler sonography. *AJR* 1995; **165:** 975–979.

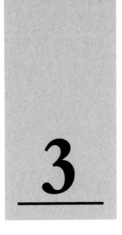

3

THE THYROID AND PARATHYROIDS

AT Ahuja

Ultrasound of the thyroid
Anatomy of the thyroid
Examination
Papillary carcinoma
Anaplastic carcinoma
Medullary carcinoma
Follicular lesion
Lymphoma
Thyroid metastases
Hurthle cell tumours
Multinodular thyroid
Thyroid cysts
Thyroiditis
Postoperative hypertrophy
Ultrasound of the parathyroids

Ultrasound of the thyroid

The patient with a thyroid nodule presents a common clinical dilemma. Clinical examination is unable to identify the true nature of the nodule, and imaging may be necessary. The aim of imaging with any modality is to distinguish a benign from a malignant lesion.

The thyroid is unique among endocrine glands in its relatively superficial location. The normally homogeneous texture of the gland, its clearly defined surrounding structures, and the proximity of constant anatomic landmarks such as the carotid artery and the internal jugular vein make it an ideal structure for evaluation by high resolution ultrasonography. Although ultrasound is sensitive in detection of thyroid nodules, in inexperienced hands it lacks specificity; this can be overcome by the fact that it is easily combined with fine-needle aspiration (FNAC) cytology. Ultrasound combined with FNAC is therefore the ideal initial investigation for thyroid nodules.

The role of ultrasound in the evaluation of thyroid nodules is well established and there are numerous reports of its use.[1,2] The aims of this chapter are:

- to familiarise the reader with the ultrasound appearances of common thyroid lesions

- to illustrate the features that help in identifying malignancy

- to show how ultrasound can demonstrate the same features that are identified by the pathologist.

Anatomy of the thyroid

This section discusses the key anatomy of the thyroid region (Figure 3.1).

The thyroid gland consists of right and left lobes connected in the midline by a narrow isthmus. The gland is surrounded by a sheath derived from the pretracheal layer of the deep fascia, which attaches the gland to the trachea and the larynx. About 10–30% of patients have a third lobe (the pyramidal lobe) arising from the isthmus, projecting upwards and running along the midline or slightly to the left, anterior to the thyroid cartilage.

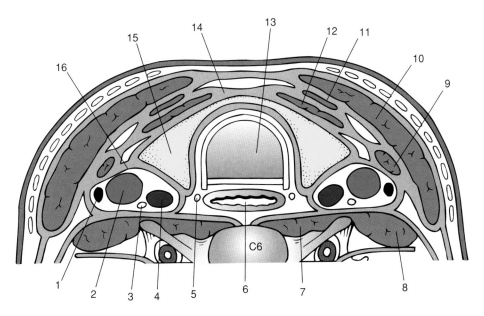

Figure 3.1 – Transverse section at the level of C6 showing relevant anatomy of the thyroid. 1. Cervical lymph node. 2. Internal jugular vein. 3. Vagus nerve. 4. Common carotid artery. 5. Recurrent laryngeal nerve. 6. Oesophagus. 7. Longus colli. 8. Scalenus anterior. 9. Omohyoid. 10. Sternocleidomastoid. 11. Sternohyoid. 12. Sternothyroid. 13. Trachea. 14. Pretracheal fascia. 15. Thyroid gland. 16. Carotid sheath.

RELATIONS OF THE LOBES

Anterior and lateral:

- strap muscles (sternohyoid and sternothyroid), which taper off towards the midline

- sternomastoid, the largest muscle of the neck, lying anterior and lateral to the strap muscles

- the superior belly of the omohyoid.

Posterior and lateral:

- carotid sheath, containing the common carotid artery (CCA), internal jugular vein (IJV), and vagus nerve

- scalenus anterior muscle.

Medial and posterior:

- larynx and trachea

- oesophagus, lying posteriorly and slightly to the left

- longus colli muscle, which is posterior and in close contact with the vertebra

- recurrent laryngeal nerve, which runs in the tracheo-oesophageal groove anterior to the longus colli.

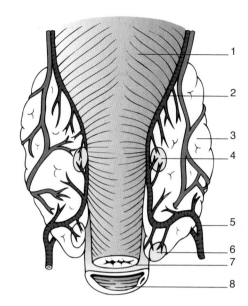

Figure 3.2 – Posterior view of the oesophagus and trachea showing the vascular relations of the thyroid and the location of the parathyroid glands. 1. Pharynx. 2. Superior thyroid artery. 3. Thyroid gland. 4. Superior parathyroid. 5. Inferior thyroid artery. 6. Inferior parathyroid. 7. Oesophagus. 8. Trachea.

RELATIONS OF THE ISTHMUS

Anterior: the strap muscles, anterior jugular vein, fascia and skin.

Posterior: the second to fourth rings of the tracheal cartilage.

BLOOD SUPPLY

The arteries to the thyroid are (Figure 3.2):

- *Superior thyroid artery:* arises from the external carotid artery and descends towards the ipsilateral thyroid lobe. At the upper pole of the gland it divides into the anterior and posterior divisions.

- *Inferior thyroid artery:* arises from the thyrocervical trunk and ascends along the back of the gland to reach its posterior surface. It is closely related to the recurrent laryngeal nerve.

- *Thyroidea ima artery:* if present, arises from the aortic arch or the brachiocephalic trunk and ascends anterior to the trachea to the isthmus.

- *Superior, middle and inferior thyroid veins:* originate from the perithyroid venous network. The superior and middle veins drain into the ipsilateral IJV, whereas the inferior thyroid vein receives tributaries from the isthmus, then anastomoses with the inferior thyroid vein from the opposite side and drains into the brachiocephalic vein.

LYMPHATICS

Lymphatic vessels from the thyroid form a subcapsular network and give rise to lateral and medial collecting trunks. These drain into the anterior and lateral chain of nodes along the IJV (deep cervical chain), and the pretracheal and paratracheal nodes.

Sonographic anatomy

The majority of structures described above can be demonstrated by high resolution ultrasound (Figure 3.3).

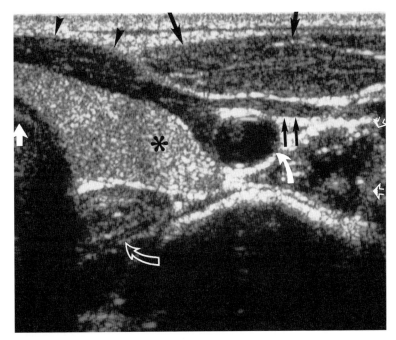

Figure 3.3 – Transverse sonogram of the left side of the neck demonstrating relevant anatomy. Bold arrow – trachea; curved white arrow – common carotid artery (CCA); open curved white arrow – oesophagus; open white arrows – scalenus anterior; black arrowheads – strap muscles; small black arrows – omohyoid muscle; large black arrows – sternocleidomastoid; asterisk – thyroid gland.

The thyroid parenchymal echoes are fine, uniform and hyperechoic compared to the adjacent muscles. The vessels within the glands are best seen at the poles. The echogenic thyroid capsule is clearly seen on ultrasound and helps to differentiate thyroid lesions from extrathyroidal masses such as parathyroid adenomas.

THYROID ULTRASOUND

1 The right lobe tends to be slightly larger than the left.
2 The lobes are often not at the same levels in the neck; this also affects the location of parathyroid lesions.
3 The base of the lobes may be quite low in the neck, at the cervicothoracic junction, and considerable hyperextension may be required for sonographic evaluation.
4 The pyramidal lobe is rarely seen due to its small anteroposterior diameter. It may be seen in the young but it undergoes progressive atrophy in adults.
5 There may be a 'pseudo-mass' at the lower pole of the thyroid gland. This 'separated' portion of the gland mimics a parathyroid lesion, particularly on transverse scans. A longitudinal scan quickly confirms its thyroid

origin (Figure 3.4). Such a mistake is common in a rounded, hypertrophied gland, as in Graves' disease or thyroiditis.
6 The oesophagus is identified as a 'bull's-eye' with an echogenic centre of air and saliva and a hypo-echoic rim because of its musculature. It is commonly deviated to the left and should not be mistaken for a mass lesion.
7 The recurrent laryngeal nerve can be seen on longitudinal scans as a thin, linear, hypo-echoic structure between the thyroid anteriorly and the longus collis posteriorly. It may have echogenic edges due to the capsule of the thyroid and the longus colli muscle.

Examination

Most of the anatomy described above can be demonstrated with high resolution transducers. However, in cases of deep-seated tumours, retrosternal/retroclavicular extension of tumours, obese patients with short necks, or patients who cannot adequately hyperextend their necks, one may have to resort to a lower resolution transducer (5 MHz, with or without a stand-off gel). The aim in these cases is to identify the relevant pathology and its major anatomical relationships.

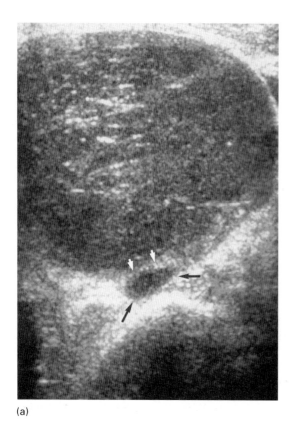
(a)

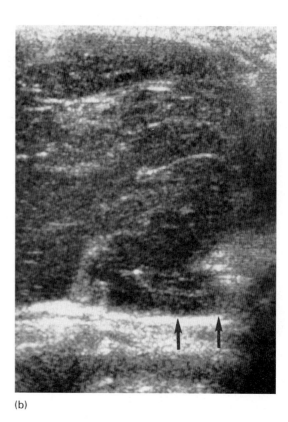
(b)

Figure 3.4 – Transverse sonogram (a) showing a hypo-echoic nodule (black arrows), separated from the thyroid by a bright thyroid capsule (white arrows). This may be mistaken for a parathyroid. However, longitudinal scan (b) shows that it is a tongue of hypertrophied thyroid gland (large black arrows).

The sonologist should start scanning in the transverse plane as the adjacent anatomical relationships of the thyroid are clearly visualised. When evaluating thyroid nodules the examination can be divided into two parts:
1 ultrasound features of the thyroid nodule
2 adjacent structures such as the carotid artery, internal jugular vein, oesophagus, strap muscles and cervical lymph nodes; examination of these structures is mandatory and forms an essential part of the evaluation of any thyroid nodule.

Ultrasound features of thyroid nodules

Before the diagnostic ultrasound appearances of various thyroid nodules are discussed, one has to be familiar with the features that can be evaluated by ultrasound, their significance, and the misconceptions (myths) that currently exist.

MULTINODULARITY

It is generally believed that malignancy is more common in a solitary nodule, and that multinodularity is usually associated with benign disease. However, ultrasound with high resolution transducers consistently demonstrates multiple clinically occult nodules which may falsely reassure the sonologist. Malignant and benign nodules are often present together in the same gland: approximately 10–20%[3,4] of papillary carcinomas may be multicentric. Thus the presence of multiple nodules within the thyroid does not indicate benignity.

SOLID/CYSTIC

It is also believed that cystic nodules are benign. However, true epithelial thyroid cysts are rare[5] and the cystic nodules seen on ultrasound invariably have a

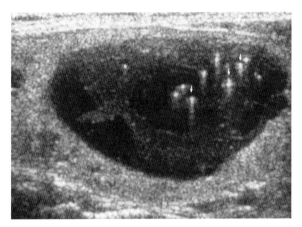

Figure 3.5 – Longitudinal sonogram demonstrating the comet tail sign (small arrows) in a colloid nodule.

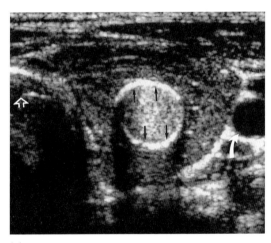

(a)

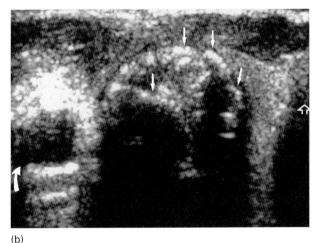

(b)

solid component. Nodules with large cystic components are usually benign nodules that have undergone cystic degeneration or haemorrhage. In the author's experience, however, almost 20–30% of papillary carcinomas also have a cystic component, indicating that not all cystic thyroid nodules are benign.

COMET TAIL SIGN

One highly specific sign of benignity of a thyroid nodule is the presence of a comet tail (Figure 3.5). In the author's experience of over 500 cases the presence of a comet tail sign invariably signified a benign colloid nodule;[6] this sign was never encountered in a malignant lesion. Aspiration usually yields viscous orange coloured fluid (consistent with colloid), and invariably requires the use of larger calibre needles.

ECHOGENICITY

It is reported that the incidence of malignancy is only 4% when a solid thyroid lesion is hyperechoic. If the lesion is iso-echoic the incidence of malignancy increases to 26%, while malignancy occurs in 63% of hypo-echoic masses.[7] In daily practice, however, benign nodules are very common and a solitary hypo-echoic nodule is statistically more likely to be benign.[4]

MARGINS

A peripheral halo of decreased echogenicity is seen around iso-/hyperechoic nodules. It is caused by either the capsule of the nodule or compressed thyroid tissue and vessels.[4] A complete halo around the lesion is 12

Figure 3.6 – Transverse sonograms showing two types of calcification associated with benign hyperplastic nodules. Note (a) the annular calcification (black arrows) in one, and (b) dense shadowing calcification in another (white arrows). Open arrow identifies the position of the trachea and curved arrow marks the CCA.

times more likely to indicate a benign lesion than a malignant lesion. If the halo is incomplete, a benign lesion is still 4 times more likely than a malignant lesion.[7] However, a halo may also be seen in 15–30% of malignancies[5,8–10] and its presence is therefore not pathognomonic of benignity.

CALCIFICATION

The presence of calcification in thyroid nodules was previously considered a sign of benignity. Calcification is detected by ultrasonography in about 10% of all thyroid nodules.[4] Peripheral rim calcification and large areas of coarse shadowing calcification are more frequently seen in benign nodules (Figure 3.6). Fine punctate calcification due to calcified psammoma bodies is seen in papillary carcinomas (25–40%).[11] Such calcification may also be seen in metastatic nodes from papillary carcinoma. Small calcific foci may be present in medullary carcinoma, both within the primary tumour and metastatic cervical nodes.[12]

COLOUR FLOW IMAGING

Colour flow imaging may be a daunting prospect to the uninitiated. There is extensive literature regarding its use in the thyroid. The author finds that the distribution of vessels within and around the nodule, rather than measurements of peak velocities, provides the best clue to the diagnosis.

There are three general patterns of vascular distribution:[13]

Type I: complete absence of flow signal within the nodule. However, in the author's experience, newer machines with their high sensitivity will invariably demonstrate small vessels within most nodules.

Type II: exclusive perinodular arterial flow signals; type II is invariably accompanied by the type I pattern.

Type III: intranodular flow with multiple vascular poles chaotically arranged, with or without significant perinodular flow.

The type III pattern is generally associated with malignant nodules, whereas types I and II are seen in benign hyperplastic nodules.[13,14]

High resolution sonography has changed the way in which thyroid nodules are evaluated. Although none of the ultrasound features above is by itself pathogno-monic for malignancy, when used in combination they are very useful in differentiating a malignant from a benign nodule.

Examination of adjacent structures

COMMON CAROTID ARTERY AND INTERNAL JUGULAR VEIN

The presence of a thrombus within the carotid artery or internal jugular vein, in association with a thyroid nodule, is a clue to the malignant nature of the nodule. Tumour thrombus, when present, is more commonly seen in follicular carcinomas and anaplastic carcinomas than in papillary carcinoma of the thyroid.[11,15]

SPREAD TO ADJACENT STRUCTURES

Involvement of the strap muscles is another clue to the malignant nature of the thyroid nodule. This is seen as loss of the normal fascial planes between the thyroid and strap muscles and ill-defined outlines of the muscle.

Extrathyroid spread, including involvement of the oesophagus, trachea, strap muscles and recurrent laryngeal nerve, is yet another clue to the malignant nature of the nodule.

CERVICAL LYMPHADENOPATHY

Although the majority of thyroid carcinomas present as a thyroid nodule, 15–30% present with an enlarged, palpable cervical lymph node.[16] Nodal metastases occur most commonly with papillary carcinomas of the thyroid, ranging from 30–40% at presentation.[17–19] Follicular thyroid carcinomas, more frequently associated with distant haematogenous metastases (lung, bone), generally exhibit a lower incidence of cervical lymphadenopathy (in the range of 10–15%).[20] The incidence of cervical metastases from well-differentiated carcinomas is far higher in patients under the age of 40 and is striking in children, where metastases are seen in 60–90% of cases.[21] The nodes commonly involved are the pretracheal and paratracheal nodes and nodes along the internal jugular vein.

Metastatic nodes from papillary carcinoma show cystic necrosis in 25% of cases and punctate calcification in 50%; they are hyperechoic relative to muscle in 80%.[22] The appearance of the metastatic node is often very similar to that of the primary tumour in the thyroid.

Although metastatic nodes from medullary carcinoma also show calcification they are invariably hypo-echoic relative to adjacent muscles.

Metastases to the thyroid, thyroid lymphoma and anaplastic carcinomas are also associated with a high incidence of adjacent nodal involvement.[11]

Now that the sonologist is familiar with evaluating the thyroid, its adjacent structures and the relevant signs that can be seen in a thyroid nodule, attention must be turned to ultrasound's primary role – the detection of malignancy. The role of ultrasound in detecting thyroid malignancy is therefore discussed next.

Papillary carcinoma

Papillary carcinoma is the most common malignancy of the thyroid, accounting for 60–70% of all thyroid malignancies.[23] The majority of patients are female, and it is the most frequent thyroid cancer in young individuals. The 20-year survival rate is reported to be as high as 90%.[11]

PATHOLOGY

The term 'occult' or 'papillary microcarcinoma' is used for lesions between 4 and 7 mm in size. Harach *et al*[24] demonstrated that 35.6% of autopsied patients in Finland had such a tumour in their thyroid and recommended that tumours less than 5 mm should be considered normal. However, most authorities believe that the malignant nature of such tumours should be recognised because nodal and distant metastases have been documented, albeit rarely.[25]

Papillary carcinomas can be located anywhere within the thyroid. They are firm, non-encapsulated or partially encapsulated tumours, and may show cystic change.

Under the microscope, psammoma bodies may be seen (40–50%)[26] in addition to the characteristic papillary nature of the tumour. Psammoma bodies are formed by infarcted papillae attracting calcium which is deposited on the dying cells. Their presence in the thyroid or adjacent nodes is pathognomonic of a papillary carcinoma.

Papillary carcinoma commonly invades regional lymphatics; this accounts for the multifocal nature of the tumour and its spread to regional nodes. Pathological

venous invasion occurs in 7% of papillary carcinomas, and anaplastic change within the tumour is rare.[26] Distant metastases to lung and bone are seen in 5–7% of cases, but survival is still prolonged, especially with radio-iodine treatment.[26] Even the presence of adjacent nodal metastases does not adversely affect the patient's prognosis.

Poor prognostic factors include:

- middle aged or elderly patient
- large size (> 3 cm)
- male sex
- vascular/extracapsular invasion
- large solid areas
- poor differentiation on pathology.

Subtypes of papillary carcinoma.

Follicular variant: usually unencapsulated, almost total follicular pattern within the tumour but with psammoma bodies and characteristic nuclei.

Diffuse sclerosing type: affects children and young adults. Tumour permeates the gland with numerous psammoma bodies and vascular and lymphatic permeation.

Encapsulated variant: 8–13% show total encapsulation; small areas of invasion may be seen within the capsule.

ULTRASOUND FEATURES

1 Predominantly hypo-echoic (77–90%).[11,14] This is due to the closely packed cell content and sparse colloid within the tumour (Figure 3.7).
2 Mostly solid (70%). However, 20–30% have a cystic component. In cystic papillary tumours with septa within, vascularity may be seen within the septa. In benign cystic modules the septa are usually avascular.
3 On ultrasound, 10–20% are multifocal.[4]
4 Punctate calcification is present in 25–40%,[11] but in some series occurs in as many as 90%.[14] Microcalcification is highly specific for papillary tumours but can also be seen in 3–5% of hyperplastic/adenomatous nodules. Typically, punctate calcification (Figure 3.7) does not exhibit posterior shadowing.
5 A halo is seen in 15–30%,[5,8–10] frequently incomplete and representing encapsulation. The remainder are ill defined with irregular outlines (Figure 3.7).

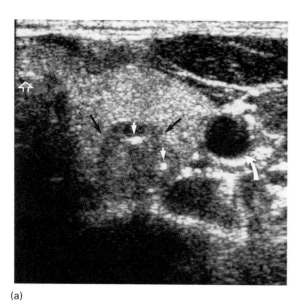
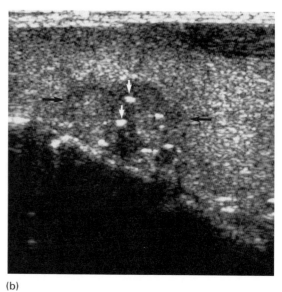

(a) (b)

Figure 3.7 – Transverse (a) and longitudinal (b) sonograms of a papillary carcinoma (black arrows). It is hypo-echoic and solid, with punctate echogenic foci (white arrows). Note that it appears well-defined on transverse scans (a), but shows irregular outlines in the longitudinal scan (b). Open arrow identifies the position of the trachea and curved arrow marks the CCA.

6 Signs of adjacent spread to strap muscles, trachea, oesophagus and recurrent laryngeal nerve may be present.

7 Characteristic adenopathy:[22]

- nodes hyperechoic relative to muscle in 80%
- distribution along cervical chain and pre/paratracheal nodes
- punctate calcification in 50% (Figure 3.8)
- cystic necrosis in 25%; in some cases the presence in the cervical chain of a thick-walled cystic mass or a cystic mass with a solid component which demonstrates vascularity on colour flow imaging (Figure 3.9) may be the only clue to the presence of an occult carcinoma in the thyroid and may be mistaken for an infected branchial cyst.[27]

8 On colour flow imaging, 90% show multiple, chaotically arranged vessels within the tumour (Figures 3.10, 3.11).[14]

Ultrasound also plays a useful role in patients who have had previous surgery for papillary cancer, as recurrences may develop:

- within the thyroid bed; the appearances of the recurrent tumour resemble primary papillary carcinoma (Figure 3.12)

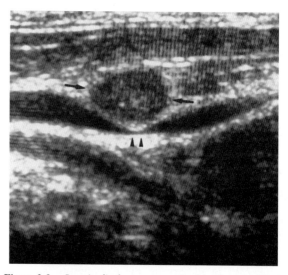

Figure 3.8 – Longitudinal sonogram of a lymph node (black arrows) with a punctate echogenic focus typical of a metastatic node from papillary carcinoma. Note its density is similar to the muscle anteriorly and the node indents the internal jugular vein (arrowheads).

- within the nodes along the cervical, pre/paratracheal chains.

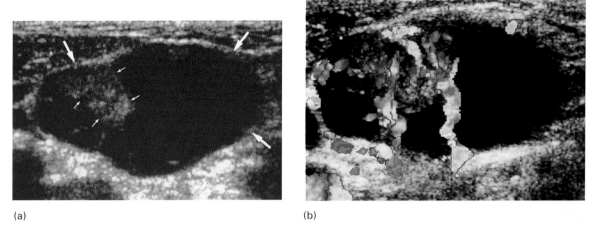

(a)   (b)

Figure 3.9 – Transverse sonogram of a large cystic metastatic node (large white arrows) from papillary carcinoma with a focal solid component (small white arrows). This cystic node may be mistaken for a branchial cyst with debris. However, note the intense vascularity within the solid component, suggesting the sinister nature of the mass.

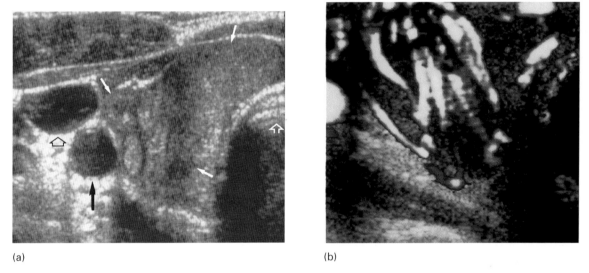

(a)   (b)

Figure 3.10 – Transverse sonogram of a papillary carcinoma seen as a solid, ill-defined heterogeneous nodule within the thyroid (white arrows). Note the marked chaotic intranodular vascularity within the nodule on colour power Doppler (b). White open arrow identifies the position of the trachea, black arrow marks the CCA and the black open arrow the IJV.

However, one must be aware of suture granulomata within the thyroid bed which may mimic tumour recurrence. These are also ill defined, solid and hypo-echoic with echogenic foci showing posterior shadowing. The echogenic foci within these lesions are usually larger and denser with greater acoustic shadowing (Figure 3.13). Ultrasound-guided fine-needle aspiration cytology readily differentiates between the two.

PAPILLARY CARCINOMA
Predominantly solid, ill-defined, hypo-echoic
Punctate calcification
Chaotic vascular pattern on colour flow imaging
Associated characteristic lymphadenopathy

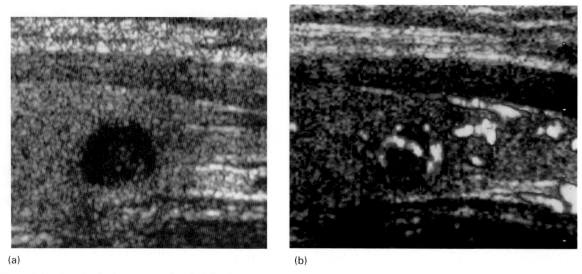

(a)   (b)

Figure 3.11 – Longitudinal sonogram of an ill-defined, hypo-echoic, heterogeneous nodule (a). The intense vascularity in such a small nodule on colour power Doppler (b) suggested the sinister nature of this nodule, a papillary carcinoma.

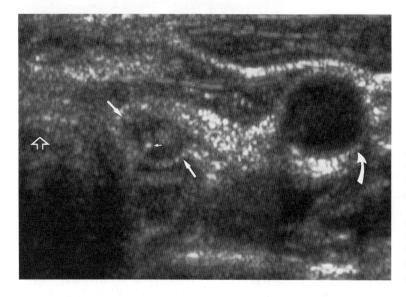

Figure 3.12 – Transverse sonogram of the thyroid bed in a patient with thyroidectomy for papillary carcinoma. Note the hypo-echoic nodule (large arrows) with a small echogenic focus (small arrows) in the thyroid bed. Appearances are of a papillary carcinoma recurrence, probably nodal. Compare this with Figure 3.13. Open arrow identifies the position of the trachea and curved arrow marks the CCA.

Anaplastic carcinoma

Anaplastic carcinoma represents 15–20%[23] of all thyroid cancers and is one of the most aggressive head and neck cancers, with survival rates of months rather than years. These tumours may represent the final stage of de-differentiation of papillary or follicular carcinomas. The diagnosis is usually clinical with a rapidly growing thyroid nodule, patients frequently presenting with pressure signs and symptoms. Ultrasound helps to confirm the clinical diagnosis and guide FNAC, which has excellent sensitivity for this tumour.

PATHOLOGY

There are two types:

- Large cell type. The commonly encountered tumour. It is frequently seen in regions of the world

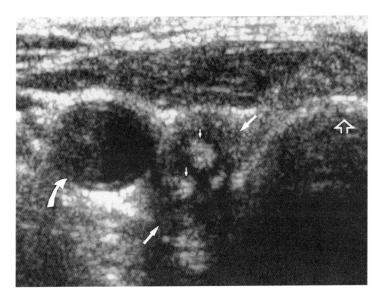

Figure 3.13 – Transverse sonogram of the thyroid bed in a patient with thyroidectomy for papillary carcinoma. Note the hypo-echoic nodule (large arrows) with large echogenic areas (small arrows) in the thyroid bed. This was a suture granuloma. Compare this with Figure 3.12. Open arrow identifies the position of the trachea and curved arrow marks the CCA.

where goitre is endemic, and represents an apparent transformation of a benign or low-grade lesion. The patients are usually elderly females, a history of goitre being present in 80%.

- Small cell carcinoma: extremely rare (its existence as an entity is often questioned).

Anaplastic carcinomas are seen as large masses with a propensity for infiltration and appear pathologically as large fleshy tumours with areas of haemorrhage and necrosis. At the periphery of the tumours, associated well-differentiated tumours may be found, representing adenomatous goitre, follicular lesions, or Hurthle cell tumours.[26]

ULTRASOUND FEATURES

1 Diffusely hypo-echoic (reflecting its closely packed cell content), often involving the entire lobe (Figure 3.14).
2 Dense amorphous calcification in 58%.[28]
3 Areas of necrosis in 78%.[28]
4 Nodal or distant metastases in 80% of patients.[15]

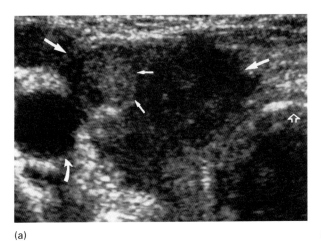

(a)

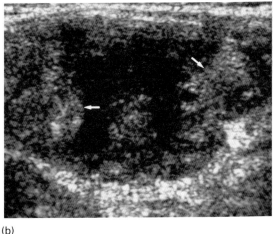

(b)

Figure 3.14 – Transverse (a) and longitudinal (b) sonograms of the thyroid showing an ill-defined, hypo-echoic mass (large arrows) against a background of nodularity (small arrows). The appearances are those of an anaplastic carcinoma. Open arrow identifies the position of the trachea and curved arrow marks the CCA.

Adjacent metastatic nodes which are often necrotic (50%).[11]

5 Adjacent vascular invasion and extracapsular spread in a third of patients.[15]

6 Frequently seen against a background of nodular goitre (47%; Figure 3.14).

7 Typically colour flow imaging shows multiple small vessels. However, necrotic tumours may be hypovascular.

> **ANAPLASTIC CARCINOMA**
> - Ill-defined, hypo-echoic, often cystic
> - Amorphous calcification
> - Background nodularity
> - Chaotic vascular pattern on colour flow imaging
> - Frequent adjacent vascular invasion
> - Frequent associated lymphadenopathy

Medullary carcinoma

Medullary carcinoma is relatively rare, representing just 5% of all thyroid cancers.[23] The tumour arises from the parafollicular C-cells which secrete thyrocalcitonin. In 10–20% of cases there is a family history of thyroid tumours or evidence of hypercalcaemia or phaeochromocytoma. In 50% nodal metastases are seen at presentation, and 15–25% have distant metastases (lung, bone, liver).[26]

PATHOLOGY

The tumour is commonly seen at the site of maximum C-cell concentration, the lateral upper two thirds of the gland.[26] It is frequently well circumscribed, but many have infiltrative borders. The tumour characteristically contains amyloid; some may show intratumoral necrosis or haemorrhage. It may also invade lymphatics and veins. In the familial forms there may be multiple intrathyroidal tumours.

ULTRASOUND FEATURES

1 Solid hypo-echoic nodule.
2 Distribution:

- focal, predominantly in the upper third of the gland in the sporadic form[23]

- multiple or diffuse involvement of both lobes is

more common in the familial form; examination of the adrenal glands is therefore mandatory.[23]

3 Echogenic foci in 80–90% of tumours, these represent both dense deposits of amyloid and associated focal calcification.[11,23] The calcification tends to be denser than in papillary carcinoma and may show frank posterior shadowing (Figure 3.15).

4 Echogenic foci seen in 50–60% of associated metastatic lymphadenopathy.[11,23] However, these nodes are hypo-echoic compared to hyperechoic nodes in papillary carcinoma.[22] Mediastinal nodes are frequently found.

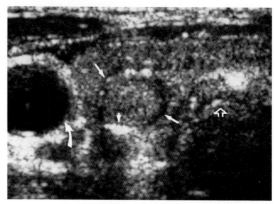

(a)

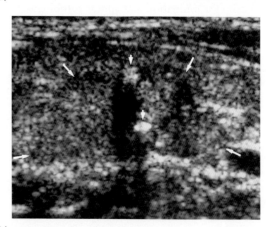

(b)

Figure 3.15 – Transverse (a) and longitudinal (b) sonograms of a medullary carcinoma (large arrows). Note that its appearance is similar to the papillary carcinoma in Figure 3.7. The echogenic foci (small arrows) are denser and exhibit posterior shadowing compared to the punctate foci in papillary carcinoma. Open arrow identifies the position of the trachea and curved arrow marks the CCA.

5 Colour flow imaging shows prominent chaotic vessels within the tumour, predominantly type III pattern.[14]

Medullary carcinoma is associated with multiple endocrine neoplasia (MEN) syndrome. These patients have a biologically aggressive tumour and may succumb to metastases earlier. The survival rate is only 55% at 5 years.[29,30]

Recurrence is common in medullary carcinoma of the thyroid. An increased serum calcitonin level is highly specific for tumour recurrence.

MEDULLARY CARCINOMA
- Solid, hypo-echoic
- Focal or diffuse
- Echogenic foci within
- Chaotic vascular pattern on colour flow imaging
- Associated characteristic lymphadenopathy

Follicular lesion

Note the use of the term 'follicular lesion' when describing follicular tumours. It is not possible by any imaging means of FNAC or core biopsy to distinguish between an invasive carcinoma and its benign counterpart (follicular adenoma). The entire specimen must be examined histologically for capsular and vascular invasion. We therefore group them under the term 'follicular lesions', and do not use the term 'adenoma'. Thus the diagnosis of a follicular lesion usually implies the need for surgical removal.

PATHOLOGY

The minimum pathological criteria for a follicular carcinoma are invasion of the capsule, or invasion through the capsule of the tumour, and invasion of the veins in or beyond the capsule. The criteria for vascular invasion apply solely to the veins in or beyond the capsule. Tumour plugs in the capillaries within the tumour have no diagnostic significance.[31]

Follicular carcinoma accounts for 2–5% of all thyroid cancers.[14] However, in iodine deficient areas these tumours are more prevalent, 25–30%.[32] When iodine is added to the diet, papillary carcinoma increases and follicular carcinomas decrease.[32] In most cases it develops from a pre-existing adenoma.[14]

There are two histological types. The differentiation is important as it affects the patient's prognosis:

1 Minimally invasive: encapsulated tumour, only invasion or penetration of the capsule but no vascular invasion.[26] These tumours rarely metastasise (8–10%),[14] and also have a low fatality rate (3%).
2 Frankly invasive: obvious vascular invasion at or beyond the level of the tumour capsule[26] and thyroid invasion. 50–80% metastasise[14] and have a high fatality rate (50%).

Both types have a propensity for haematogenous spread to bone, lung, brain and liver, and patients frequently present with distant metastases. Nodal metastases are relatively uncommon.

ULTRASOUND FEATURES (FOLLICULAR LESION)

1 Predominantly solid. If present, the cystic portion is frequently small.
2 Homogeneous in 70% (Figure 3.16).
3 Commonly hyperechoic (Figure 3.16). Hypoechoic lesions are relatively uncommon.
4 Calcification is rare.
5 Haloed in 80%.
6 On colour flow imaging, the majority (80–90%) of benign follicular lesions show perinodular blood flow signals (type II; Figure 3.17), whereas malignant follicular lesions have a type III vascularity in over 90% of cases.[14]

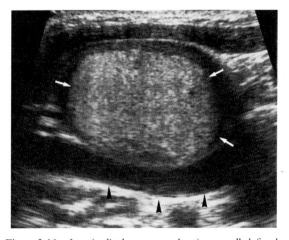

Figure 3.16 – Longitudinal sonogram showing a well-defined, homogeneous, solid, hyperechoic thyroid nodule (arrows), suggesting a follicular lesion. Note that it indents the CCA (arrowheads) but does not invade it.

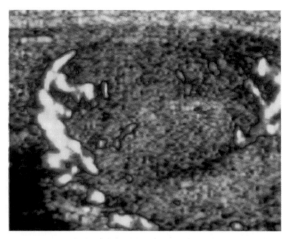

Figure 3.17 – Colour power Doppler of a homogeneous, iso-echoic, well-defined solid nodule showing predominantly perinodular vascularity. Following surgery this was confirmed to be a follicular adenoma.

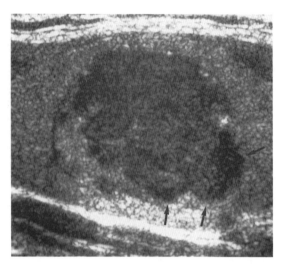

Figure 3.18 – Longitudinal sonogram of the thyroid showing a solid, heterogeneous, predominantly hypo-echoic nodule with ill-defined edges (arrows), suggesting its malignant nature. This patient presented with bone metastases and the thyroid nodule was confirmed to be a follicular carcinoma.

FOLLICULAR LESION
- Hyperechoic, homogeneous
- Haloed
- Calcification is rare
- Chaotic vascular pattern on colour flow imaging in follicular carcinoma

---

As stated earlier, it is not possible by any imaging technique, or FNAC cytology, to distinguish early invasive carcinoma from its benign counterpart. Follicular carcinomas are associated with hyperplastic/adenomatous thyroid nodules in 60–70% of cases.[14] Identification of such a nodule within a multinodular thyroid is difficult and ultrasound may be unable to identify these foci of malignancy.

However, the diagnosis of malignancy can be suggested on ultrasound if any nodule is ill defined and hypo-echoic with heterogeneous internal echoes (Figure 3.18). Further signs suggesting malignancy include: a thick irregular capsule; profuse chaotic, tortuous perinodular and intranodular vessels; vascular invasion and extra capsular spread.

Lymphoma

Lymphoma may arise primarily from the thyroid or involve the thyroid secondarily as part of a systemic lymphoma. Primary and secondary involvement of the thyroid by lymphoma is rare, accounting for only 1–3% of all thyroid malignancy. Non-Hodgkin's lymphoma is more common than Hodgkin's disease, and an antecedent history of Hashimoto's thyroiditis is almost always present.[11,23] It affects elderly women, often presents as a rapidly enlarging mass, and may extend outside the thyroid gland.

PATHOLOGY

Lymphomatous involvement of the thyroid may be focal or diffuse. Invasion beyond the thyroid into muscles and soft tissues is seen in 50–60% of cases[33,34] and vascular invasion in 25%.[35]

ULTRASOUND FEATURES
1 The thyroid is commonly hypo-echoic. However, lymphoma may sometimes present as simple glandular enlargement with no obvious abnormality in the thyroid echopattern (associated characteristic lymphadenopathy may be the only clue).
2 Lymphoma may appear as focal or diffuse abnormality within the gland (Figures 3.19, 3.20).

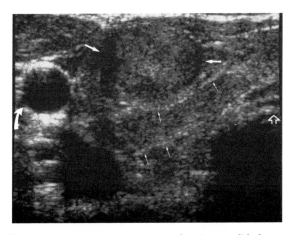

Figure 3.19 – Transverse sonogram showing a solid, hypo-echoic lymphomatous nodule (large white arrows) in the thyroid. Note the hypo-echoic, heterogeneous parenchyma with thin fibrotic streaks (small white arrows) suggesting a background of Hashimoto's thyroiditis. Open arrow identifies the position of the trachea and curved arrow marks the CCA.

3 Focal lymphomatous nodules may have a 'pseudocystic' appearance with posterior enhancement and may be mistaken for cystic lesions (the gain settings must be increased to identify the solid nature of the nodule).

4 A heterogeneous echopattern may be seen in diffuse lymphomatous involvement.[23] In such cases the differential diagnosis includes anaplastic carcinoma and thyroid metastases (Figure 3.20).

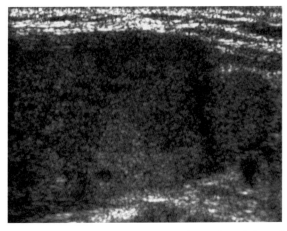

Figure 3.20 – Longitudinal sonogram of an enlarged thyroid with a hypo-echoic, heterogeneous echopattern of diffuse lymphomatous involvement. A similar appearance may also be seen in metastatic thyroid involvement.

5 Colour flow imaging is non-specific as the nodules may be hypovascular or may demonstrate a chaotic (type III) pattern.

6 Associated large, round, hypo-echoic, hypervascular lymph nodes which demonstrate posterior enhancement are characteristic. These nodes may displace the major vessels but rarely cause thrombosis.[23]

LYMPHOMA
- Hypo-echoic
- Focal or diffuse thyroid involvement
- Pseudocystic appearance
- Heterogeneous echopattern
- Changes of Hashimoto's thyroiditis
- Non-specific vascularity on colour flow imaging
- Associated characteristic lymphadenopathy

Thyroid metastases

Metastases to the thyroid are infrequent, occurring late in the course of the disease and generally as the result of spread by a haematogenous (more commonly) or lymphatic route. Its incidence, in patients with a known primary is 2–17%. Common sites of origin include: melanoma 39%, breast 21%, renal cell carcinoma 10%.

PATHOLOGY

The lesions are often solitary and well circumscribed with an appearance similar to that of the primary tumour.[26] The gland may however show diffuse involvement, without the formation of a nodule.

ULTRASOUND FEATURES[36]

1 Large and solid, predominantly in the lower pole (Figure 3.21).

2 Homogeneously hypo-echoic mass.

3 Non calcified.

4 Typically, well defined (Figure 3.21).

5 Invariably associated with adjacent malignant cervical nodes or disseminated disease with liver, bone or lung metastases.

(a) 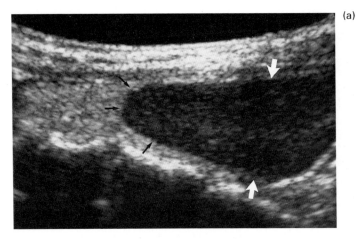 (b)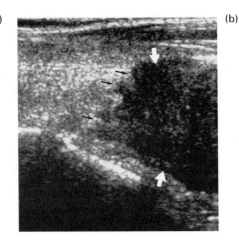

Figure 3.21 – Longitudinal sonograms of the thyroid showing solid, hypo-echoic large metastatic nodules (white arrows) in the lower poles. The edges may be well defined (a) or less commonly ill defined (b).

6 Heterogeneous echopattern seen in diffuse thyroid involvement.
7 Colour flow imaging may show increased vessels or may be unremarkable.

THYROID METASTASES
- Large and solid focal mass
- Homogeneously hypo-echoic mass
- Typically well defined
- Diffuse heterogeneous echopattern
- Non-specific vascular pattern on colour flow imaging
- Invariably associated with disseminated disease

Hurthle cell tumours

Hurthle cells are derived from follicular epithelium. They can be found in a number of conditions and cannot be considered specific for any disease entity. They are seen in multinodular thyroid, chronic thyroiditis, Hashimoto's thyroiditis and long-standing hyperthyroidism. Most Hurthle cell lesions are follicular in pattern, and so the criteria for differentiating between benign and malignant are similar to those for follicular lesions (capsular and vascular invasion). Their ultrasound appearances may also closely resemble a follicular lesion.

Previously considered benign, these tumours do exhibit a potential for malignancy and may metastasise to the lungs and lymph nodes (30%). They are uncommon lesions and bridge the gap between benign and malignant thyroid nodules.

The pathological criteria for malignancy are met more frequently in Hurthle cell tumours as compared to their non-Hurthle counterparts. Thus, whereas only 2–3% of solitary, encapsulated tumours show invasive characteristics, 30–40% of Hurthle cell lesions show such features.[26]

PATHOLOGY

Most Hurthle cell neoplasms are solitary mass lesions that show complete or partial encapsulation. They may rarely undergo tumour infarction (particularly after FNA). There are two definite pathological types, benign and malignant. Lesions greater than 4 cm frequently (80%) exhibit malignant criteria.

ULTRASOUND FEATURES

1 Mixed internal echogenicity, i.e. they have hypo-echoic and hyperechoic components within the same nodule (Figure 3.22).
2 They are often ill defined and show an incomplete halo around the lesion.
3 Mostly solid.
4 No evidence of calcification.

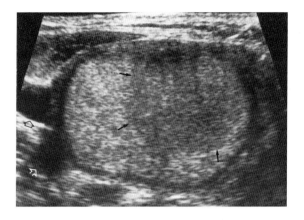

Figure 3.22 – Transverse sonogram showing a well–defined, pre-dominantly hyperechoic nodule with areas of hypo-echogenicity within (arrows). At surgery this was found to be a Hurthle cell adenoma. Note its similarity to a follicular lesion. White open arrow marks the CCA and the black open arrow identifies the IJV.

5 Colour flow imaging is non-diagnostic as the appearances are similar to a follicular lesion, i.e. the nodule may show intranodular vascularity, type III pattern.
6 Presence of adjacent malignant nodes may be the only clue to their malignant nature.

HURTHLE CELL TUMOUR
- Commonly resembles a follicular lesion on ultrasound
- Mixed internal echogenicity (hyperechoic and hypo-echoic)
- Incomplete halo
- Non-specific vascular pattern on colour flow imaging

Having considered the malignant tumours of the thyroid, we must now address the more common benign nodules. In daily practice, malignant thyroid lesions are uncommon, whereas benign thyroid nodules are ubiquitous. The commonest condition encountered in thyroid ultrasound practice is a multinodular thyroid.

Multinodular thyroid

'Multinodular goitre' is a common term used to describe multiple nodules within the thyroid. The term 'goitre' implies an enlarged gland, so what does one call a normal sized thyroid containing multiple nodules? We therefore do not encourage the use of the term 'multinodular goitre' but prefer to call these glands 'a multinodular thyroid'.

It is the commonest (80%) pathological condition of the thyroid: 2–6% of the population have a clinically palpable mass.[26] The patients are frequently asymptomatic but may present with compressive symptoms or a rapidly enlarging mass (the commonest cause of which is haemorrhage within a nodule).

PATHOLOGY

Hyperplastic nodules are composed of brown thyroid tissue. Fibrosis and calcification are noted within. Microscopically, colloid lakes alternating with normal to hyperplastic foci of thyroid tissue, haemorrhage, fibrosis and calcification are found. A variable amount of lymphocytic infiltration may also be seen.

The initiating event is proliferation involving one or a group of follicles. The adjacent follicles are quiescent. Vascular compression (due to follicular hyperplasia) leads to focal ischaemia, necrosis and inflammatory changes. Progression of the disease first leads to macronodule formation with a solid structure but subsequently changes such as haemorrhage, fibrosis and calcification take place.[26] As these changes are occurring, the gland remains under hormonal influence. The follicular and vascular distortion interferes with distribution of iodide and thyrotropin, resulting in areas of focal hyperplasia (which receive excess thyrotropin) and areas of atrophy (due to thyrotropin deficiency).

ULTRASOUND FEATURES

1 Solid nodules are frequently iso-echoic, with a small percentage of hypo-echoic nodules (5%).
2 Well-defined margins. The nodules are unencapsulated; the halo is composed of compressed thyroid and adjacent vessels.
3 Cystic component in 60%. This may represent haemorrhage or colloid within the nodule. Haemorrhage into a nodule is the commonest cause of a rapidly enlarging thyroid mass.
4 Heterogeneous internal echopattern with multiple septa, solid and cystic portions (Figure 3.23).
5 Calcification in 25%. The end stage of a hyperplastic nodule is calcification, which may be curvilin-

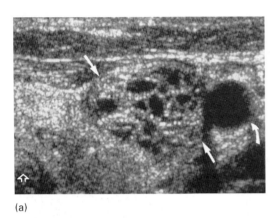

(a)

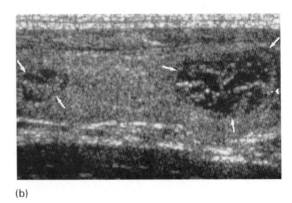

(b)

Figure 3.23 – Transverse (a) and longitudinal (b) sonograms showing typical appearances of hyperplastic/adenomatous nodules (arrows). Note the cystic/colloid spaces and intervening septa. Open arrow identifies the position of the trachea and curved arrow marks the CCA.

ear, annular or dysmorphic calcification within the gland. The calcification may be seen as large, densely calcified areas with posterior shadowing (Figure 3.6).

6 Comet tail sign (Figure 3.5), signifying the presence of colloid within a nodule, is commonly seen in multinodular thyroid.

7. On colour flow imaging the nodules either show type I, or a type II pattern (Figure 3.24). If the nodule becomes toxic it may demonstrate intranodular vascularity (type III pattern). Debris (clots) within

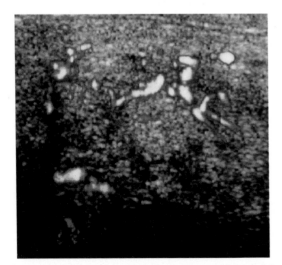

Figure 3.24 – Colour power Doppler showing peri/intranodular vascularity within an iso-echoic hyperplastic nodule.

haemorrhagic nodules are avascular, the septa within the nodules are also avascular. The presence of vascularity within the debris and septa should raise the possibility that the nodule may not be a hyperplastic nodule (Figure 3.25). FNAC for such a nodule is mandatory.

Most pathologists use the term 'hyperplastic nodules' to describe the nodules found in a multi-nodular thyroid. However, some pathologists may use the term 'adenomatous nodules', which can create confusion. An adenomatous nodule is a distinct and separate entity from a follicular adenoma. For sonologists (and many pathologists) distinction between whether a nodule is an adenomatous nodule or a hyperplastic nodule is academic, they represent the same benign lesion found in a multi-nodular thyroid.

While some authors may state that differentiation between adenomatous nodules and hyperplastic nodules is possible on ultrasound, there is no point in wasting time and energy in trying to differentiate between the two. Keep things simple and use the term 'hyperplastic nodule' whenever possible!

How can one identify or exclude the presence of malignancy within such a gland? If there is a nodule with the obvious features of malignancy as described earlier, FNAC readily confirms the diagnosis. But if there are no typical features of malignancy seen, should one perform FNAC? How does one then identify which nodule to biopsy? The decision as to whether or not to perform a FNAC when malignancy is not suspected must be

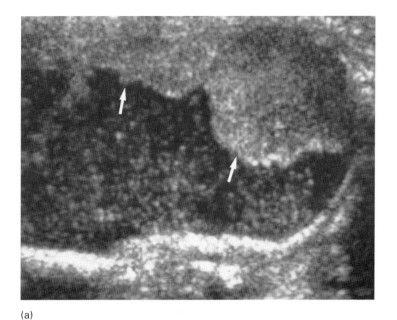

(a)

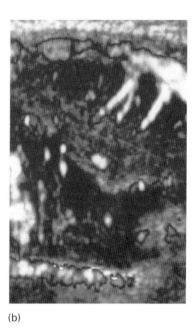

(b)

Figure 3.25 – Longitudinal sonograms (a, b) of a thyroid nodule with a cystic component with internal debris and a lobulated iso-echoic component anteriorly. Colour power Doppler (b) demonstrates large vessels within the solid component. At surgery this was found to be a follicular carcinoma.

guided by local practice. In many centres, the largest (dominant) nodule is aspirated in order to rule out a frankly malignant lesion.

There will always be a small group of patients, however, where the presence of malignancy is missed. It is detected only after surgery or when the patient presents some time later with obvious clinical and sonographic signs of malignancy. This is a recurring problem that still cannot be overcome. The only reassurance is that the incidence of malignancy in such a thyroid is extremely low, only 1–3%.[11]

MULTINODULAR THYROID
- Multiple nodules
- Frequently iso-echoic, well defined
- Solid and cystic elements
- Comet tail sign
- Florid calcification
- On colour flow imaging they exhibit type I and type II pattern

---

Thyroid cysts

True epithelial thyroid cysts are rare.[5] Most cystic thyroid lesions are due to haemorrhage or degeneration within a hyperplastic nodule. The ultrasound appearances of these have been discussed.

Thyroiditis

Patients with thyroiditis may present with a palpable thyroid nodule. The common types of thyroiditis encountered in clinical practice are Hashimoto's thyroiditis, de Quervain's subacute thyroiditis and acute suppurative thyroiditis.

Hashimoto's thyroiditis

Hashimoto's thyroiditis is the most common of the chronic thyroiditides,[37] it is more common in women and has a peak incidence between 40 and 60 years of age. The diagnosis is usually based on serology as it is an auto-immune condition. Hypothyroidism is present at presentation or develops later in 50% of cases.[11]

There is an associated increased risk for the development of non-Hodgkin's lymphoma.[38] Hashimoto's thyroiditis may be associated with other auto-immune conditions.

ULTRASOUND APPEARANCES

Acute:

- Focal nodular thyroiditis; small, hypo-echoic, avascular nodules with ill-defined outlines. These represent areas of lymphocytic infiltration and may be mistaken for a mass lesion (micronodular pattern).

- Diffuse thyroiditis; multiple nodules with a micronodular pattern involving the whole gland. The gland is avascular.

Chronic: enlarged gland with lobulated outline and multiple ill-defined hypo-echoic areas separated by echogenic fibrous septa (Figure 3.26). The gland is hypervascular (mainly arterial) both within the parenchyma and the fibrous septa (Figure 3.27).[14] The appearances are similar to the 'thyroid inferno' seen in Graves' disease.[39] This hypervascularity in chronic thyroiditis when hypothyroidism develops is due to the hypertrophic action of TSH. Following treatment (when the TSH levels return to normal) the hypervascularity decreases.[39]

Atrophic, end stage: small atrophic avascular gland with heterogeneous echoes (Figure 3.28).

de Quervain's subacute thyroiditis

The patient characteristically presents with neck pain, fever and lethargy shortly after an upper respiratory tract illness or viral disease. The region of the thyroid is painful. In the acute stage the patient may be thyrotoxic, followed by progress to a hypothyroid state in 2–4 months; typically, after six months of onset of pain, the patient returns to a euthyroid state.[37,40]

ULTRASOUND FEATURES

In the *acute state* the patient presents with a painful, palpable nodule.
1 The 'nodule' is usually focal, ill defined, hypo-echoic and subcapsular in location (Figure 3.29).
2 There is no associated calcification.
3 There is no halo.
4 The adjacent thyroid echoes are heterogeneous.
5 Pressure on the lesion usually elicits pain. There may be adjacent inflammatory nodes.

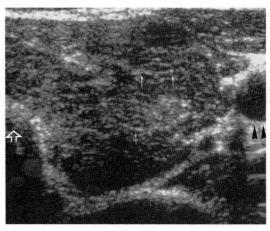

(a)

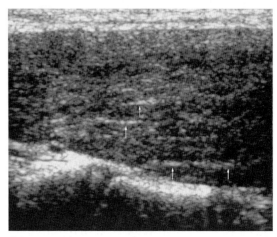

(b)

Figure 3.26 – Transverse (a) and longitudinal (b) sonograms of the thyroid showing diffuse enlargement, hypo-echoic heterogeneous echopattern with bright fibrotic streaks (white arrows). Appearances are of Hashimoto's thyroiditis. Open arrow identifies the position of the trachea and arrowheads mark the CCA.

6 On colour flow imaging these focal hypo-echoic areas are avascular; the rest of the gland may show normal or diminished vascularity (due to oedema).[14]

In the *subacute phase* the entire lobe, and even the contralateral lobe, is diffusely hypo-echoic with enlargement of the gland. The gland remains painful and adjacent inflammatory nodes are still seen.

Six months after the onset of pain the ultrasound appearance of the gland usually returns to normal. However,

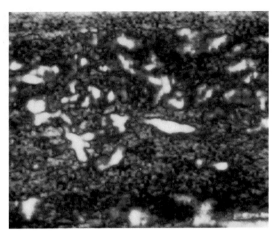

Figure 3.27 – Colour power Doppler showing marked vascularity within the thyroid in Hashimoto's thyroiditis.

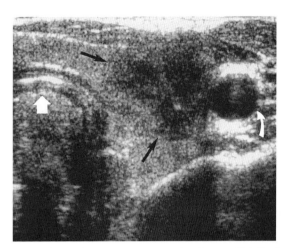

Figure 3.29 – Transverse sonogram showing an ill-defined, hypo-echoic nodule in the thyroid anteriorly (black arrows). The patient presented with fever and pain over the thyroid. The diagnosis of thyroiditis was confirmed by FNAC. White arrow identifies the position of the trachea and curved arrow marks the CCA.

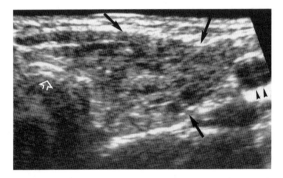

Figure 3.28 – Transverse sonogram showing a small, post-Hashimoto's, atrophic heterogeneous thyroid gland (arrows). Open arrow identifies the position of the trachea and arrowheads mark the CCA.

in some cases there is nodule formation[23] or there may be atrophy of the thyroid.[41]

The role of ultrasound in these patients is to assess the evolution of the disease. Patients usually recover with medical treatment within six months, however the prognosis is worse if the hypo-echoic regions continue to increase in size while the patient is receiving treatment.

Acute suppurative thyroiditis

Acute suppurative thyroiditis, although rare, particularly affects children. It has a left-sided predominance and is frequently associated with a fourth branchial cleft anomaly. The child typically presents acutely with pain, thyroid swelling, fever, and pain on swallowing. There is usually a history of previous similar episodes.

ULTRASOUND FEATURES

The infection usually begins in the perithyroidal soft tissues. The thyroid gland itself is relatively resistant to infection because it has a thick fibrous capsule, is very vascular and contains a high iodine content and extensive lymphatics.

Both intra- and extrathyroid abscesses are seen as ill-defined, hypo-echoic, heterogeneous mass with internal debris with or without septa and gas. Adjacent inflammatory nodes are frequently present.

In cases where the infection involves only the perithyroidal tissues, the fascial planes between the thyroid and the soft tissues are maintained (Figure 3.30). When the thyroid is secondarily involved, the fascial planes are obliterated and the extension of the abscess into the thyroid is clearly seen (Figure 3.31).

The role of ultrasound is to confirm an abscess, involvement of the thyroid gland (if any), and the relationship of the abscess to the major neck vessels.[42] The abscess can be aspirated at the same time, under ultrasound guidance. Ultrasound is also used to monitor the

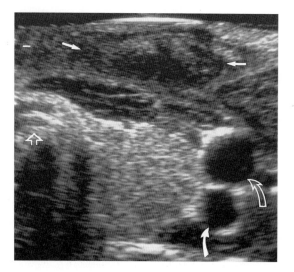

Figure 3.30 – Transverse sonogram showing a small, heterogeneous collection (arrows) anterior to the strap muscles, not involving the thyroid. Open arrow identifies the position of the trachea, curved arrow marks the CCA and the curved open arrow the IJV.

response to treatment. A barium study is indicated to identify the pyriform fossa sinus which is usually associated with acute suppurative thyroiditis.

Postoperative hypertrophy

Patients who have had surgery often present later with a palpable 'nodule' in the thyroid region. In most patients who have undergone surgery for benign thyroid nodules (hyperplastic), the cause of the enlargement is probably a recurrent nodule or residual nodule. In such cases ultrasound is useful as it can evaluate the nature of the nodule.

In those who have undergone surgery for Graves' disease, however, the palpable nodule may represent hypertrophy of the residual thyroid tissue rather than a true nodule.

On ultrasound, regenerating thyroid gland after surgery for Graves' disease is hypo-echoic, with rounded contours and a heterogeneous echopattern (Figure 3.32). It is centred in the region of the thyroid bed and often superficial in location, thus presenting as a palpable thyroid 'nodule'. On colour flow imaging there is vascularity within the 'nodule'; however there is no displacement or chaotic arrangement of the vessels.

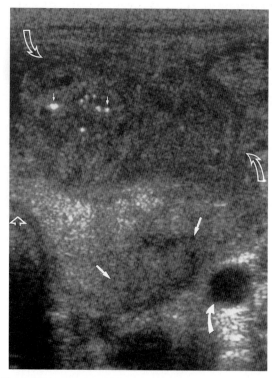

Figure 3.31 – Transverse sonogram showing a heterogeneous collection (curved open arrows) with an intrathyroidal component (large arrows) of the abscess. Note the pocket of gas within the collection (small arrows). Open arrow identifies the position of the trachea and curved arrow marks the CCA.

Conclusion

The primary role of ultrasound in a case of thyroid nodule should always be the detection of malignancy. Ultrasound is also an effective triage in the management of patients with a thyroid nodule. It identifies three categories of patients:

1 Those with thyroid malignancy who will benefit from surgery.
2 Those in whom surgery may be unnecessary or detrimental, e.g. patients with thyroiditis, multinodular thyroid.
3 Patients who may either avoid surgery or have their surgery delayed. This group primarily includes those with follicular lesions. The management of these patients depends on local practice. This may include surgery in the first instance or a 'wait and see' policy.

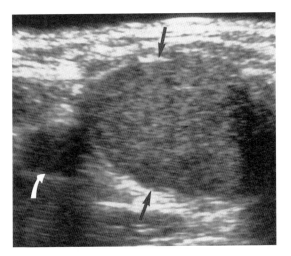

Figure 3.32 – Transverse sonogram showing a rounded, hypo-echoic, hypertrophic thyroid gland (black arrows) following surgery for Graves' disease. Curved arrow identifies the CCA.

Ultrasound of the parathyroids

The main indication for imaging of the parathyroid glands is localisation of tumoral lesions causing hyper-parathyroidism. Pathologically, the three main aetiologies are: adenoma, which is almost always limited to a single gland; hyperplasia, which affects all four glands; and carcinoma, which, like adenoma, involves only one gland. Adenoma is the cause of primary hyper-parathyroidism in 80% of cases, hyperplasia in less than 20% and carcinoma in 1%.[43]

The indications for parathyroid imaging can be controversial as is the choice of imaging modality. The aim of this section is to familiarise the sonologist with the ultrasound, appearances of parathyroid lesions and the common mistakes one may make during scanning.

Is pre-operative parathyroid localisation necessary?

There is dispute about the routine use of pre-operative imaging in the localisation of parathyroid adenomas. In many institutions, in a patient not previously operated on for parathyroid disease, pre-operative localisation is not carried out. This decision is based on the fact that operative time, morbidity and mortality are not influenced by pre-operative localisation of parathyroid adenomas for hyperparathyroidism.[44,45] The surgical procedure in these institutions consists of bilateral perithyroidal exploration, particularly at the inferior poles where parathyroid adenomas are common. In experienced hands the success rate is over 90%.[46–49] In fact, some recommend that the only localisation required is that of a good parathyroid surgeon.[46]

However, some surgeons may request localisation pre-operatively, suggesting that this reduces both operative time and the risk of operative damage to the recurrent laryngeal nerve and normal parathyroids.[50,51] These surgeons will perform a unilateral neck exploration if the pre-operative imaging is definitive, but will convert to bilateral surgery if the imaging findings are equivocal or multifocal abnormality is shown.

In patients with a previous failed exploration, secondary explorations have only a 70–80% success rate,[52] and there is little dispute that localisation should be attempted prior to reoperative parathyroidectomies or prior to a parathyroidectomy in a patient who has had a previous thyroidectomy.[53] In these situations the gland is more likely to be in an ectopic position.

Anatomy and technique

Although the majority of people have four glands – two pairs at the upper and lower poles of the thyroid gland – 25% of individuals have more than this number.[54,55] The superior glands are more constant in position along the dorsal aspect of the superior pole of the lateral thyroid lobes, near the recurrent laryngeal nerve. The inferior glands are more varied in position along the dorsal aspect of the inferior poles of the thyroid gland. However, they may be some distance away from the lower poles of the thyroid, at the cervicothoracic junction or even in the superior mediastinum.

The following paragraphs discuss the typical and atypical locations[56] of parathyroid lesions.

TYPICAL SITES OF A PARATHYROID LESION

Superior: behind the upper and middle third of the thyroid gland.

Inferior:

● behind the lower pole of the thyroid

● behind the strap muscles

● within the thyro-thymic ligament (1–2 cm away from the lower pole of the thyroid).

ATYPICAL SITES OF A PARATHYROID LESION

Undescended: glands along the common carotid artery.[57,58] They are similar in appearance to nodes at this site. The internal vascularity and FNA may help to distinguish the two.

Intrathyroidal: in the middle to lower third of the thyroid gland. The intrathyroid glands are aligned in the long axis of the thyroid. They mimic thyroid nodules and are difficult to diagnose.

Retrotracheal: these glands are difficult to detect because of acoustic shadowing from the trachea. If they are large, they protrude across the midline and can then be visualised.

In our experience it is easiest to start scanning in the transverse plane, beginning above the level of the upper pole of the thyroid and moving downwards scanning through the thyroid to the level of the clavicle. It is mandatory to use a 7.5–10 MHz transducer. The patient lies supine with the neck hyperextended, as false negative scans may be obtained in patients who are incorrectly positioned, particularly in elderly patients who may be unable to hyperextend the neck. Parathyroid adenomas are often located low in the neck; hyperextension elevates these lesions into the neck where they are easily visualised. In patients with short necks, or obese patients with thick necks, it may be necessary to use a lower frequency transducer (5 MHz) with a stand-off gel block to improve visualisation.

A few points to note:

- In our experience we have been unable to identify and locate normal parathyroid glands with confidence, even with 12 MHz transducers.

- Parathyroid lesions are separated from thyroid tissue by an echogenic plane between the two, representing the capsule around the thyroid and parathyroid.

- Irrespective of the nature of the lesion, abnormal glands are frequently hypo-echoic compared to the thyroid. This is due to the uniform hypercellularity of the lesions.[56]

- In 15–20% there are variations in the appearance of the lesion. Some glands may be iso-echoic to the thyroid gland, and some may contain obvious cystic change, septa and debris (due to cystic/haemorrhagic degeneration).

- Calcification is rare in adenomas but more common in carcinomas and hyperplasia due to secondary hyperparathyroidism. [56]

A parathyroid lesion may be confused with normal anatomic structures such as:

- longus colli, oesophagus, blood vessels

- nodes, particularly those related to the recurrent laryngeal nerve and sometimes even nodes along the carotid artery and internal jugular vein.

- thyroid nodules may be mistaken for a parathyroid lesion.

COLOUR FLOW IMAGING

Colour flow imaging is routinely used to localise and evaluate a parathyroid lesion and to differentiate it from other lesions such as a lymph node. The following points should be noted with regard to parathyroid lesions: [56]

- Most parathyroid lesions (90%) demonstrate a hypervascular pattern (Figure 3.33).

- 10% are avascular. This is a feature of lesions less than 1 cm in diameter, deep-seated lesions and those with cystic necrosis.

- The vascularity is intraparenchymal, mainly arterial (Figure 3.33).

- The only perinodular flow is at the hilum. This is located at the caudal part of the inferior glands and at the cranial part of the superior glands.

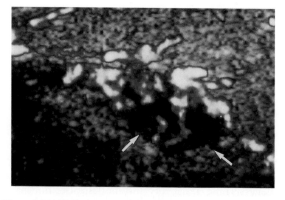

Figure 3.33 – Colour power Doppler showing intraparenchymal vascularity within a parathyroid adenoma (arrows).

Ultrasound features

PARATHYROID ADENOMA

1 Parathyroid adenomas appear as oval sonolucent masses (Figure 3.34).

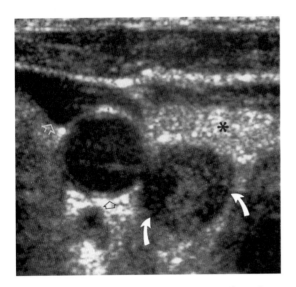

Figure 3.34 – Transverse sonogram showing a round, sonolucent parathyroid adenoma (curved arrows), posterior to the thyroid (asterisk). Black open arrow identifies the CCA and white open arrow the IJV.

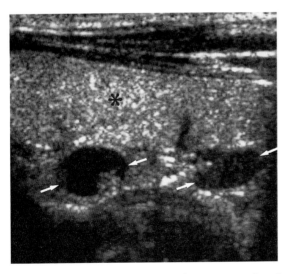

Figure 3.35 – Longitudinal sonogram showing two enlarged, oval parathyroid glands (arrows) posterior to the thyroid (asterisk).

2 Retrothyroid lesions tend to be oval or flat (Figure 3.35), since the parathyroid glands in this position develop within longitudinally aligned fascial planes and are clearly separated from the thyroid by a well-defined echogenic line.[43] Infrathyroid lesions are generally spherical. [43]
3 Calcification is rare.
4 Lesions may have a cystic component (Figure 3.36). Multiple small cysts are more common than a single large cyst. [43]
5 Sonographic pattern alone cannot differentiate a benign from a malignant lesion. Benign lesions are mobile when the patient swallows whereas malignant lesions may be fixed. [43]
6 Intrathyroid parathyroid adenomas occur in 1–2%; they have no specific features, are usually hypo-echoic and well defined with a very sharp edge between the adenoma and the adjacent thyroid parenchyma, [43] and show parenchymal vascularity within.

PARATHYROID HYPERPLASIA

Parathyroid hyperplasia tends to be more spherical than adenomas and may show the presence of calcification.

PARATHYROID CARCINOMA

The ultrasound appearances in parathyroid carcinoma are similar to those in parathyroid adenoma, except that there may be demonstrable invasion of adjacent structures plus immobility on swallowing. Metastases to adjacent nodes are seen in 21–28% of cases.[59]

PARATHYROID CYSTS

Parathyroid cysts:

● are more frequently seen in women than men

● may be present in the neck or anterior mediastinum

● may, when large, compress the oesophagus, trachea and recurrent laryngeal nerve

● 95% of cases occur below the level of the inferior thyroid border; 65% involve inferior parathyroid glands[59]

● are well defined and thin walled; the cyst fluid has high parathormone but low T3 and T4 levels.

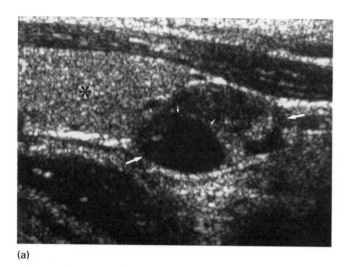
(a)

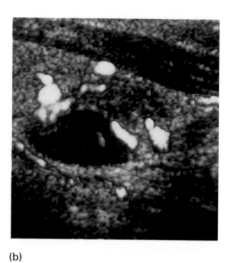
(b)

Figure 3.36 – Longitudinal sonogram (a) showing a parathyroid adenoma (large arrow) with a cystic component (small arrows) below the lower pole of the thyroid (asterisk). Note the vascularity within the solid component on colour power Doppler (b).

ETHANOL ABLATION

Ethanol ablation of a parathyroid adenoma is performed under ultrasound guidance by percutaneous injection. It is used in patients with primary or secondary hyperparathyroidism who may be poor surgical candidates. This technique was first described by Solbiati *et al*[60] and is now a commonly performed procedure.[61] It is indicated only in patients with not more than two enlarged glands, neither exceeding 2–2.5 cm in maximum diameter.

The procedure is performed under ultrasound control, care being taken to avoid over-penetration and leakage of the sclerosant around the recurrent laryngeal nerve. Injection of absolute alcohol is accompanied by a rapid disappearance of flow signal within the enlarged gland. The procedure is terminated when flow signals are no longer seen within the injected gland.[56]

The most common complication is recurrent laryngeal nerve palsy following the injection. Its incidence is higher in inexperienced hands and is frequently due to over-penetration before injecting alcohol. As the needle is withdrawn into the lesion, a track is created and alcohol leaks through this track.

Recurrences following ablation may be caused by proliferation of parathyroid tissue within the fibrotic gland, or the development of a new hyperplastic gland (in 30% of cases).[56]

The choice of initial imaging modality (if any) in hyperparathyroidism will always be governed by local practice and expertise. This section has described the useful ultrasound features that help in identifying parathyroid adenomata and hyperplastic glands. While discussion of the merits of other foms of imaging in parathyroid disease is beyond the scope of this text, there is no doubt that ultrasound can be a cost-effective initial means of imaging. It also has a useful role as an adjunct to other imaging methods (e.g. Sestamibi isotope studies) and in the treatment (i.e. ethanol ablation) of certain groups of patients.

References

The thyroid

1. Watters DAK, Ahuja AT, Evans RM. Role of ultrasound in the management of thyroid nodules. *Am J Surg* 1992; **164:** 654–657.

2. King AD, Ahuja AT, Metreweli C. The role of ultrasound in the diagnosis of a large, rapidly growing, thyroid mass. *Postgrad Med J* 1997; **73(861):** 412–414.

3. Woolner LB, Beahs OH, Black BM *et al.* Classification and prognosis of thyroid cancer. *Am J Surg* 1961; **102:** 354–387.

4. McIvor NP, Freeman JL, Salem S. Ultrasonography of the thyroid and parathyroid glands. *ORL* 1993; **55:** 303–308.

5. Simeone JF, Daniels GH, Mueller PR *et al.* High resolution real time sonography of the thyroid. *Radiology* 1982; **145:** 431–435.

6. Ahuja A, Chick W, King W, Metreweli C. Clinical significance of the comet tail artifact in thyroid ultrasound. *J Clin Ultrasound* 1996; **24**: 129–133.

7. Solbiati L, Giangrande A, De Pra L et al. Percutaneous injection of parathyroid tumours and ultrasound guidance: treatment for secondary hyperparathyroidism. *Radiology* 1985; **155**: 607–610.

8. Solbiati L, Volterrani L, Rizzatto G et al. The thyroid gland with low uptake lesions: evaluation with ultrasound. *Radiology* 1985; **155**: 187–191.

9. Propper RA, Skolnick ML, Weinstein BJ, Dekker A. The non-specificity of the thyroid halo sign. *J Clin Ultrasound* 1980; **8**: 129–132.

10. Noyek AM, Finkelstein DM, Kirsch JC. Diagnostic imaging of the thyroid gland. In: Falk SA, ed. *Thyroid disease: Endocrinology, Surgery, Nuclear Medicine, and Radiotherapy.* New York: Raven Press, 1990; pp 79–126.

11. Yousem DM, Scheff AM. Thyroid and parathyroid. In: Som PM, Curtin HD, eds. *Head and Neck Imaging,* 3rd edn. St Louis: Mosby, 1996; pp 952–975.

12. Gorman B, Charboneau JW, James EM et al. Medullary thyroid carcinoma: role of high resolution ultrasound. *Radiology* 1987; **162**: 147–150.

13. Lagalla R, Cariso G, Midiri M, Cardinale AE. Echo–Doppler couleur et pathologie thyroidienne. *J Echograph Med Ultrasons* 1992; **13**: 44–47.

14. Solbiati L, Livraghi T, Ballarati E, Ierace T, Crespi L. Thyroid gland. In: Solbiati L, Rizzatto G, eds. *Ultrasound of Superficial Structures.* London: Churchill Livingstone, 1995; pp 49–85.

15. Compagno J. Diseases of the thyroid. In: Barnes L, ed. *Surgical Pathology of the Head and Neck.* New York: Marcel Dekker, 1985; pp 1435–1486.

16. McQuone SJ, Eisele DW. Cervical lymph node metastases in well-differentiated thyroid carcinoma. *Proceedings 4th International Conference on Head and Neck Cancer,* 1996; 967–971.

17. Noguchi M, Yamada H, Ohta N et al. Regional lymph node metastases in well-differentiated thyroid carcinoma. *Int Surg* 1987; **72**: 100–103.

18. Mazzaferri EL, Young RL. Papillary thyroid carcinoma: a ten year follow up report of the impact of therapy in 576 patients. *Am J Med* 1981; **70**: 511–518.

19. Carcangiu ML, Zampi G, Pupi A et al. Papillary carcinoma of the thyroid: a clinicopathologic study of 241 cases treated at the University of Florence, Italy. *Cancer* 1985; **55**: 805–828.

20. Harness JK, Thompson NW, McLeod MK et al. Follicular carcinoma of the thyroid gland: trends and treatment. *Surgery* 1984; **96**: 972–980.

21. Frankenthaler RA, Sellin RV, Cangir A et al. Lymph node metastases from papillary-follicular thyroid carcinoma in young patients. *Am J Surg* 1990; **160**: 341–343.

22. Ahuja AT, Chow L, Chick W et al. Metastatic cervical nodes in papillary carcinoma of the thyroid: ultrasound and histological correlation. *Clin Radiol* 1995; **50**: 229–231.

23. Bruneton JN, Normand F. Thyroid gland. In: Bruneton JN, ed. *Ultrasonography of the Neck.* Berlin: Springer-Verlag, 1987; pp 22–50.

24. Harach HR, Fransilla KO, Wasenius V. Occult papillary carcinoma of the thyroid: a normal finding in Finland. A systematic autopsy study. *Cancer* 1985; **56**: 531–538.

25. Patchefsky AS, Keller IB, Mansfield CM. Solitary vertebral column metastasis from occult sclerosing carcinoma of the thyroid gland. *J Clin Pathol* 1970; **53**: 596–601.

26. LiVolsi VA. Pathology of thyroid disease. In: Falk SA, ed. *Thyroid disease: Endocrinology, Surgery, Nuclear Medicine and Radiotherapy.* Lippincott-Raven, Philadelphia, 1997; pp 65–104.

27. Ahuja A, Ng CF, King W, Metreweli C. Solitary cystic nodal metastasis from occult papillary carcinoma of the thyroid mimicking a branchial cyst: a potential pitfall. *Clin Radiol* 1998; **53**: 61–63.

28. Takashima S, Morimoto S, Ikezoe J et al. CT evaluation of anaplastic thyroid carcinoma. *AJR* 1990; **154**: 1079–1085.

29. Kaufman FR, Roe TF, Isaacs H, Weitzman JJ. Metastatic medullary carcinoma in young children with mucosal neuroma syndrome. *Pediatrics* 1982; **70**: 263–267.

30. Norton JA, Froome BA, Farrell RE, Wells SA. Multiple endocrine neoplasia Type IIb: the most aggressive form of medullary carcinoma. *Surg Clin North Am* 1979; **59**: 109–118.

31. Lang W, Choritz H, Hundeshagen H. Risk factors in follicular thyroid carcinomas. A retrospective follow up study covering a 14 year period with emphasis on morphological findings. *Am J Surg Pathol* 1986; **10**: 246–255.

32. Williams ED, Doinach I, Bjanarson O, Michie W. Thyroid cancer in a iodide rich area. *Cancer* 1977; **39**: 215–222.

33. Anscombe AM, Wright DH. Primary malignant lymphoma of the thyroid – a tumour of mucosa associated lymphoid tissue: review of seventy-six cases. *Histopathology* 1985; **9**: 81–87.

34. Burke JS, Butler JJ, Fuller LM. Malignant lymphomas of the thyroid. *Cancer* 1977; **39**: 1587–1602.

35. Oertel JE, Heffess CS. Lymphoma of the thyroid and related disorders. *Semin Oncol* 1987; **14**: 333–342.

36. Ahuja A, King W, Metreweli C. Role of ultrasonography in thyroid metastases. *Clin Radiol* 1994; **49**: 627–629.

37. Price DC. Radioisotopic evaluation of the thyroid and the parathyroids. *Radiol Clin North Am* 1993; **31(5)**: 991–1015.

38. Takashima S, Ikezoe J, Morimoto S et al. Primary thyroid lymphoma: evaluation with CT. *Radiology* 1988; **168**: 765–768.

39. Lagalla R, Caruso G, Benza I, Novara V, Calliada F. Echo-Colour Doppler in the study of hypothyroidism in adults. *Radiol Med* (in Italian) 1993; **86**: 281–283.

40. Schwartz SI, Shires GT, Spencer FC et al. *Principles of Surgery,* 3rd edn. New York: McGraw Hill, 1979; p 1547.

41. Gooding GA. Sonography of the thyroid and parathyroid. *Radiol Clin North Am* 1993; **31(5)**: 967–989.

42. Ahuja AT, Griffiths JF, Roebuck DJ et al. The role of ultrasound and oesophagography in the management of acute suppurative thyroiditis in children associated with congenital pyriform fossa sinus. *Clin Radiol* 1998; **53**: 209–211.

The parathyroids

43. Moreau JF. Parathyroid glands. In: Bruneton JN, ed. *Ultrasonography of the Neck*. Berlin: Springer-Verlag, 1987; pp 51–63.

44. Carlson GL, Farndon JR, Clayton B *et al*. Thallium isotope scintigraphy and ultrasonography: comparative studies of localisation techniques in hyperparathyroidism. *Br J Surg* 1990; **77(3):** 327–329.

45. Miller DL. Pre-operative localisation and international treatment of parathyroid tumours: when and how? *World J Surg* 1991; **15(6):** 706–715.

46. Thompson CT. Localisation studies in patients with hyperparathyroidism. *Br J Surg* 1988; **75:** 97–98.

47. Edis AJ, Sheedy PF, Beahrs OH *et al*. Results of reoperation for hyperparathyroidism, with evaluation of preoperative localisation studies. *Surgery* 1978; **84:** 384–391.

48. Reading CC, Charboneau JW, James EM *et al*. High resolution parathyroid sonography. *AJR* 1982; **139:** 539–546.

49. Satava RM, Beahrs OH, Scholz DA. Success rate for cervical exploration for hyperparathyroidism. *Arch Surg* 1975; **110:** 625–627.

50. Russell CF, Laird JD, Ferguson WR. Scan-directed unilateral cervical exploration for parathyroid adenoma: a legitimate approach. *World J Surg* 1990; **14(3):** 406–409.

51. Levin KE, Clark AH, Duh Qy *et al*. Reoperative thyroid surgery. *Surgery* 1992; **111(6):** 604–609.

52. Attie JN. Localization procedures for parathyroid disease. *Proceedings 4th International Conference on Head & Neck Cancer*, Vol IV, 1996: 405–411.

53. van Heerden JA, James EM, Karsell PR *et al*. Small part ultrasonography in primary hyperparathyroidism. Initial experience. *Ann Surg* 1982; **195:** 774–779.

54. Livolsi V. In: Sternberg SS, ed. *The Thyroid and Parathyroid: Diagnostic Surgical Pathology,* 2nd edn. New York: Raven, 1994; pp 523–560.

55. Livolsi V. Pathology of the parathyroid glands. In: Barnes L, ed. *Surgical Pathology of the Head and Neck*. New York: Marcel Dekker, 1985; pp 1487–1563.

56. Fugazzola C, Bergamo AI, Andreis I, Solbiati L. Parathyroid glands. In: Solbiati L, Rizzatto G, eds. *Ultrasound of Superficial Structures*. London: Churchill Livingstone, 1995; pp 87–114.

57. Doppman JL, Shawker TH, Krudy AG *et al*. Parathymic parathyroid: CT, US and angiographic findings. *Radiology* 1985; **157:** 419–423.

58. Fraker DL, Doppman JL, Shawker TH *et al*. Undescended parathyroid adenoma: an important etiology for failed operations for primary hyperparathyroidism. *World J Surg* 1990; **14:** 342–348.

59. Yousem DM, Scheff AM. Thyroid and parathyroid. In: Som PM, Curtin HD, eds. *Head and Neck Imaging*, 3rd edn. St Louis: Mosby, 1996; pp 952–975.

60. Solbiati L, Giangrande A, De Pra L *et al*. Percutaneous injection of ethanol of parathyroid tumours under ultrasound guidance: treatment for secondary hyperparathyroidism. *Radiology* 1985; **155:** 607–610.

61. Karstrup S, Transbol I, Holm HH, Glenthog A, Hegedus L. Ultrasound guided chemical parathyroidectomy in patients with hyperparathyroidism: a prospective study. *Br J Radiol* 1989; **62:** 1037–1042.

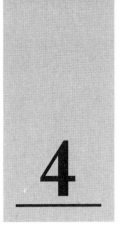

4

LYMPH NODES

RM Evans

Anatomy
Ultrasound anatomy
Classification systems
Criteria of malignancy

Introduction

In the normal adult neck there may be up to 300 lymph nodes, ranging in size from 3 mm to 3 cm. It is an understatement to say that the anatomy and its various associated classifications, groupings, subgroupings and, more recently, levels, is complex. The radiologist who decides to ignore the subtleties and complexities of the lymphatics of the head and neck region will not be alone. Yet, if one wishes to examine the head and neck region, one cannot ignore the lymphatic system. Many pathologies in the head and neck region present as a palpable lymph node. Most cervical lymph nodes are within 1–2 cm of the skin surface, and the superior resolution of ultrasound now allows the morphology and blood flow characteristics of lymph nodes to be clearly defined. Its resolution is superior to anything that computed tomography (CT) or magnetic resonance imaging (MRI) can currently offer.

Anatomy

Lymph nodes are small, oval or reniform bodies, typically 0.1–2.5 cm long, lying in the course of lymphatic vessels. There is usually a small indentation on one side, the hilum, through which blood vessels enter and leave and from which the efferent lymphatic also emerges (Figure 4.1). Multiple afferent lymphatics drain into the outer cellular cortex of the node; lymph then enters a labyrinth of lymphatic channels within the node.

Macrophages line these channels or are entangled within the fibres crossing them. Lymph is exposed to these phagocytic cells and also to the activities of B- and T-lymphocytes adhering to the endothelia. These vessels form a dense subcapsular plexus which initially drains into the subcapsular sinus (Figure 4.1). From the subcapsular sinus multiple radial cortical sinuses lead to the medulla, coalescing as larger medullary sinuses. The medullary sinuses or lymphatic cords have a parallel arrangement at the medulla as they converge to form the large efferent vessel leaving the node.

The vasculature of the lymph node mirrors its physiological activity. Intranodal vessels are sparse within the medulla. In the cortex, arteries form dense arcades of arterioles and capillaries in numerous anastomosing loops, eventually returning to multiple branching vessels and veins. Capillaries are particularly prominent around the follicles of the cortex, while venules are found in large numbers in the paracortical zones, providing an important site of lymphocytic migration.

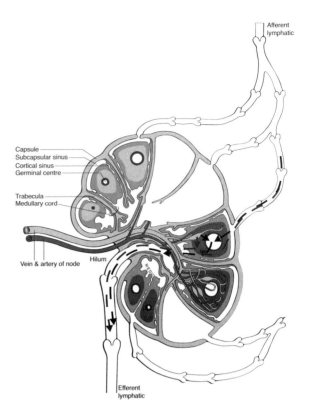

Figure 4.1 – Lymph node anatomy.

When a node undergoes antigenic stimulation, it reacts with an increase in size and vascularity. The number and size of germinal centres within the follicles increase as lymphocytes and macrophages proliferate. The numerous plasma cells in the medulla undergo differentiation. This is mirrored by an increase in vascularity within the node, the density of the capillary beds in the outer cortex greatly increasing.[1]

Our understanding of the human lymphatic system owes a great deal to Rouviere's original work.[2] The lymphatic system consists of a series of valved vessels with lymph nodes distributed along the course of vessels. Flow is controlled by valves, however the flow can be reversed by tumour or infection. In the head and neck, flow tends to be in a caudal direction towards either the right lymphatic duct or the thoracic duct on the left (Figure 4.2). Shunting can occur when a lymph node contains a metastasis, either to ipsilateral nodes or possibly to a node in the contralateral neck.

Many classification systems have evolved following on from Rouviere's work. As in other aspects of radiol-

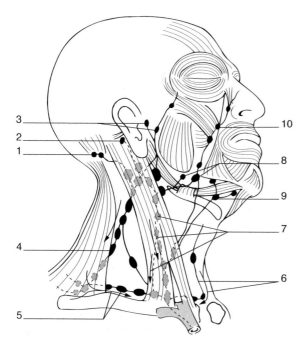

Figure 4.2 – Rouviere's original schematic representation of the lymphatic chains of the neck. 1. Occipital nodes. 2. Mastoid nodes. 3. Parotid nodes. 4. Spinal accessory lymphatic chain. 5. Transverse cervical lymphatic chain. 6. Anterior jugular lymphatic chain. 7. Internal jugular lymphatic chain. 8. Submaxillary nodes. 9. Submental nodes. 10. Facial node.

ogy, it is important that the radiologist, surgeon and physician speak the same language. It is essential to use a common classification system and to have a knowledge of the various terms; for clarification a glossary of the terms and alternative terms used in describing lymph nodes is given in Table 4.1.

Ultrasound anatomy

Where does the beginner start when trying to evaluate the lymph nodes of the neck? A simple reproducible system is required for examining the neck. This section will describe such a system; for each area examined, the anatomy of the lymph nodes will be discussed in detail.

A standard examination consists of a series of 'sweeps' by the probe (numbered 1–10, Figure 4.3), starting in the submental region and extending over one side of the neck. If the system is followed on the other side of the neck, the majority of the cervical lymph node territories will have been covered.

Submental region (Figure 4.4)

The probe is held transversely. Identify the two heads of the anterior belly of the digastric muscles as they come off the back of the symphysis mentis of the mandible. The floor of the submental triangle is the mylohyoid muscle. Sweep the probe down to the

Table 4.1 – Terms and alternative terms used in describing lymph nodes

Common terms	Alternative terms/description
Jugulodigastric node	'Sentinel' (highest) node of internal jugular chain
Deep cervical chain	Internal jugular chain
	Lateral cervical chain
Omohyoid node	Deep cervical chain lymph node just superior to omohyoid (where it crosses jugular vein)
Virchow's node	'Signal' node
	Lowest node of deep cervical chain
Transverse cervical chain	Supraclavicular chain
Troisier's node	Most medial node of transverse cervical chain – can be involved in carcinoma of the stomach
Spinal accessory chain	Posterior triangle chain
	Dorsal cervical chain
	Superficial cervical chain
Anterior cervical chain	Includes prelaryngeal, pretracheal and paratracheal nodes
Pretracheal nodes	Delphian node – important in carcinoma of the larynx.
Paratracheal nodes	Recurrent laryngeal nodes
Retropharyngeal nodes	Lateral nodes are nodes of Rouviere

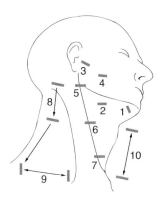

Figure 4.3 – Cervical ultrasound examination.

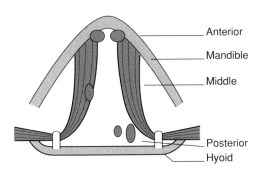

Figure 4.4 – Submental region.

hyoid bone, looking superficial to the mylohyoid and between the digastric muscles. Nodes are commonly seen anteriorly behind the mandible in the midline between the digastric muscle insertions. More inferiorly, nodes may be seen on, or just medial to, the digastric muscles. These nodes are occasionally asymmetrical in distribution with a cluster of nodes seen on one side only. Rarely, nodes are seen clustered near the hyoid bone in the inferior aspect of the submental region. The number of nodes found in the submental area varies from one to eight. Normally, in an adult there are between one and three nodes. Submental nodes tend to have an elliptical or slightly rounded shape.

These nodes receive lymph from the chin, lips, cheeks, floor of mouth and anterior tongue. They in turn drain into the submandibular nodes and then the upper deep cervical chain.

Submandibular region (Figure 4.5)

The probe is now swung around to one side of the patient, with the patient's head turned to the opposite side. The key to assessing the submandibular region is the submandibular gland itself. Scanning parallel to the plane of the body of the mandible and angling the probe cranially, the submandibular gland is identified posterior to the anterior belly of the digastric muscle. The posterior free border of the mylohyoid muscle can be seen indenting the anterior aspect of the gland. Nodes are described in relation to the submandibular gland. Use the submandibular gland as a reference point and comment on whether the node is anterior, superior, or posterior to the gland. There are usually between three and six nodes (average four) in the submandibular region. As elsewhere in the neck, their size varies in inverse proportion to the number of nodes present.

Small nodes are constantly seen anterior to the submandibular gland between the mandible and the digastric muscle on ultrasound. Superiorly, nodes are also detected flanking the facial artery. Nodes may also be present posterior to the submandibular gland. Rarely, nodes may lie deep to the posterior aspect of the gland.

The submandibular gland undergoes early encapsulation during its embryonic development, therefore the majority of submandibular nodes are true extraglandular nodes. Very occasionally a subcapsular lymph node may be present. Although these subcapsular nodes are in intimate contact with the parenchyma they are not true intraglandular nodes. The vast majority of submandibular nodes lie outside the submandibular gland (as distinct from the parotid region, which will be discussed later).

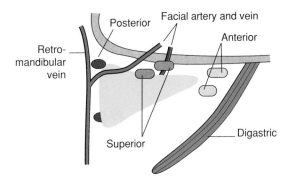

Figure 4.5 – Submandibular region.

The submandibular nodes drain the anterior facial structures and skin as well as the floor of mouth and anterior oral cavity. They predominantly drain into the deep cervical chain.

Parotid region (Figure 4.6)

Unlike the submandibular gland the parotid gland undergoes encapsulation late in its embryonic development. Lymph nodes are thus incorporated both deep to the capsule (subcapsular) and within the parenchyma of the gland itself (predominantly within the superficial lobe) during its embryological development. Parotid nodes may therefore be present superficial to the gland (i.e. extraparotid), subcapsular (extraglandular) or lying deep within the parenchyma of the gland (intraglandular).

The parotid region must be scanned both transversely and coronally. With the parotid gland as the point of reference, care must be taken to examine the area between the posterior parotid and the ear. In this region the superficial parotid or pre-auricular nodes are found (extraparotid nodes). Three or four small nodes (particularly in the infant) can be found anterior to the tragus. Subfascial nodes are usually found at two sites: anterior to the tragus (pre-auricular node) and posteriorly within the tail of the gland. There are usually one or two subcapsular pre-auricular nodes and possibly up to three or four subcapsular infra-auricular nodes in the tail of the parotid. They are commonly identified with ultrasound in children. The deep nodes, i.e. intraglandular nodes, lie within the superficial lobe and in the fascia between superficial and deep lobes. A cluster of nodes may be present near the external carotid artery and where the retromandibular vein leaves the parotid to join the external jugular vein.

The area primarily drained by the parotid nodes is the skin of the forehead, temporal regions and external auditory canal. In addition lymph drains from the Eustachian tube, buccal mucosa, posterior cheek and gums into parotid nodes. These nodes in turn drain into the deep cervical chain.

Facial region (Figure 4.7)

If the probe is moved anteriorly from the anterior aspect of the superficial lobe of the parotid, along a line drawn to the corner of the mouth, one will be in the buccal region. If facial nodes are present they should be found in this region. Facial nodes tend to be very small nodes and are rarely encountered in ultrasound. They are subcutaneous and generally lie along the plane of the facial artery and vein. There are two main groups: the inferior maxillary group and the buccinator or buccal group. The inferior maxillary nodes are found along the anterior border of the masseter. The most inferior node of this group may lie on the inferior border of the mandible; the patient can often feel this node if it is enlarged as it is rolled over the bony mandible. The buccal nodes lie in the fat pad anterior to the masseter muscle and superficial to the buccinator muscle.

The facial nodes drain the area from the lids to the upper lips; they then drain into the submandibular nodes.

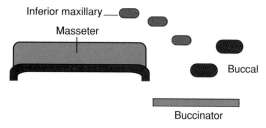

Figure 4.7 – Facial region.

Deep cervical chain (Figure 4.8)

The deep cervical or jugular chain of lymph nodes forms the main lymphatic thoroughfare of the neck. It is a vertical lymphatic escalator extending from the level of the digastric muscle to the root of the neck.

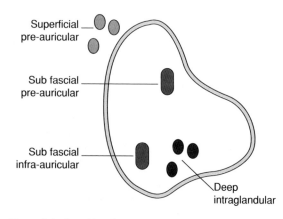

Figure 4.6 – Parotid region.

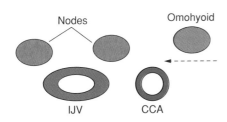

Figure 4.8 – Deep cervical chain.

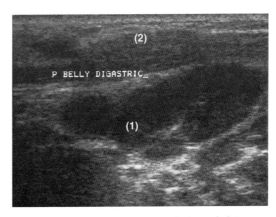

Figure 4.9 – Benign jugulodigastric node (1) underlying posterior belly of digastric muscle. Note parotid superiorly (2).

The key to assessing the deep cervical chain is to scan the internal jugular vein (IJV), transversely from the level of the tail of the parotid to its junction with the subclavian vein. Just as in scanning the deep veins of the leg, compression is important. Always 'bounce' the probe along the IJV. This does three things: it allows identification of the IJV, it maintains the IJV in the centre of the probe, and it ensures that you do not miss a thrombosed IJV (a not uncommon state when extensive metastatic lymphadenopathy is present). Nodes will be readily identified adjacent to the IJV, predominantly arranged around its anterolateral aspect.

The deep cervical chain is divided into upper, middle and lower sections by the hyoid bone and cricoid cartilage, although the latest AJCC[3] (1997) classification uses the cricothyroid membrane, and not the cricoid cartilage, as the level for dividing the deep cervical chain into mid and lower regions. Nodes in the upper part of the deep cervical chain abut the posterior belly of the digastric muscle (Figure 4.9). The largest node is the most superior – the jugulodigastric (JD) node. This is often orientated along the line of the digastric rather than the IJV, occasionally having a significant kink as it lies back behind the posterior belly of the digastric. It can be difficult to differentiate between the JD node and the posterior belly of the digastric. Identification of the digastric muscle is done quite easily by angling the probe obliquely across the tail of the parotid, identifying the posterior belly as it runs obliquely from deep to the sternomastoid down to the hyoid.

Another key muscle to identify is the omohyoid muscle. This comes down off the lateral portion of the body of the hyoid to cross the common carotid artery near its mid point. When bulky, the omohyoid can easily be mistaken for a lymph node as it crosses from medial to lateral anterior to the common carotid artery.

Rotating the probe to a sagittal plane to confirm the anatomy usually solves the problem. As the omohyoid then takes off more laterally across the neck, it marks a fairly constant lymph node landmark – the supra-omohyoid node, which is anterior to the IJV just superior to the omohyoid muscle.

Rouviere[2] described two subgroups of lymph nodes making up the deep cervical chain: a lateral and an anterior chain. The lateral group forms a garland of nodes around the lateral border of the IJV. As it extends inferiorly, the lateral chain swings medially behind the IJV. The anterior group are extensive in number superiorly, occupying the space between the digastric muscle superiorly and lying directly anterior to the IJV. There may be up to five nodes superiorly in the adult; however, in children, up to ten nodes may be present. More inferiorly the supra–omohyoid node lies in the mid portion. Distally, nodes directly anterior to the IJV are rare.

If one considers the right deep cervical chain, nodes are typically found between the ten o'clock and two o'clock positions (Figure 4.10). Passing inferiorly, nodes rotate laterally, so they are found in the nine o'clock moving to six o'clock position. Examining the left neck, the nodal distribution represents a mirror image. Note that the nodes lying medial to the common carotid artery are not deep cervical or jugular chain in origin; they are paratracheal chain nodes.

The deep cervical nodes receive lymph from the parotid, retropharyngeal and submandibular nodes. Inferiorly they empty into the IJV or subclavian vein, or drain directly into the thoracic duct on the left or

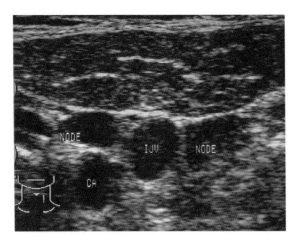

Figure 4.10 – Malignant left mid cervical nodes at the ten o'clock and two o'clock positions. IJV, internal jugular vein; CA, carotid artery.

the right lymphatic duct on the right, which empties into the junction of the IJV and subclavian vein.

Posterior triangle (Figure 4.11)

The posterior triangle or spinal accessory chain forms a triangle with the deep cervical chain and transverse cervical chain inferiorly. Superiorly the spinal accessory chain blends with the deep cervical chain, and one cannot differentiate between the two at the apex of the triangle.

As its name implies, the lymph node chain follows the spinal accessory (XI) nerve. Rouviere[2] described one or possibly two parallel rows of nodes accompanying the spinal accessory nerve in his original dissections. In order to cover the course of the accessory chain one needs to remember the landmarks of the XI nerve. It

emerges from the skull base via the jugular foramen. It then passes posteriorly deep to the posterior belly of the digastric and sternocleidomastoid muscles to run into the posterior triangle before dipping behind the anterior border of trapezius. A line drawn from the mastoid tip to the acromion represents the course of the spinal accessory nerve. The operator should scan transversely from the mastoid along the predicted line of the spinal accessory nerve. Remember that the XI nerve is a superficial structure sitting on the fascial carpet of the posterior triangle. Look for the plane between the sternomastoid and the underlying scalene and levator scapulae muscles as nodes will be identified in this superficial plane, i.e. within 1–2 cm of the skin surface. One can safely ignore the structures deep to the scalene muscles. Inferiorly, pick out the anterior border of trapezius; this effectively marks the junction of the posterior triangle chain and the transverse cervical chain.

The point where the sternomastoid muscle overlies the posterior belly of the digastric marks the junction of the spinal accessory and the deep cervical chains. One cannot differentiate between the two at this point.

The spinal accessory chain drains occipital and mastoid nodes, parietal scalp, lateral neck and shoulder lymphatics. It then drains primarily into the transverse cervical chain.

Transverse cervical chain (Figure 4.12)

Once the acromion is reached, the probe can be turned through 90° into a sagittal plane. If one keeps the bottom of the probe aligned on the clavicle and sweeps medially towards the sternal notch, one will be scanning along the plane of the transverse cervical vessels, i.e. the plane of the transverse cervical (supraclavicular) lymph node chain. In practice this means scanning with the inferior aspect of the probe on (or in most cases just above) the clavicle, looking to identify the subclavian vessels more medially. When the probe reaches the sternomastoid, the jugulo-subclavian junction should be identified. This point marks the junction of the transverse cervical chain and the deep cervical chain. The most medial node of the transverse cervical chain is known as Troisier's node as he was the first to point out that this node may become invaded in carcinoma of the stomach.

The transverse cervical chain receives lymph from the spinal accessory chain, deep cervical chain, upper anterior chest wall and the skin of the anterolateral neck.

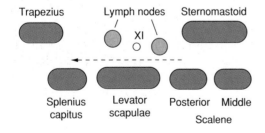

Figure 4.11 – Posterior triangle.

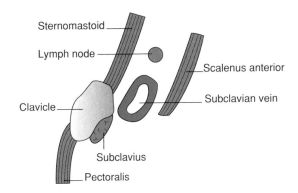

Figure 4.12 – Transverse cervical chain.

Anterior cervical nodes (Figure 4.13)

Now take the probe back to the midline and pick out the hyoid bone. This is the starting point for examining the anterior cervical nodes. Scanning transversely from the hyoid, sweep inferiorly to identify the thyroid cartilage of the larynx, cricoid, trachea, thyroid isthmus and then trachea again before it disappears into the mediastinum – the anterior cervical region will then have been covered.

This group is divided into four subgroups:

Prelaryngeal nodes

Rarely enlarged, the so-called 'Delphian node' sits in front of the cricoid membrane. It signals subglottic involvement in carcinoma of the larynx.

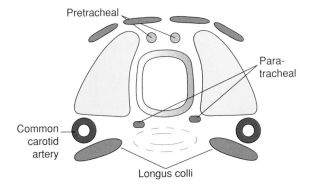

Figure 4.13 – Anterior cervical nodes.

Prethyroid nodes

Rouviere[2] describes one or two pre-isthmus nodes as a common finding in his dissections. These are rarely identified on ultrasound.

Pretracheal nodes

The pretracheal nodes are superficial nodes following the course of the anterior jugular vein, anterior to the trachea, below the thyroid. They drain the thyroid gland and lymph from the muscles and skin of the anterior neck. They drain into the thoracic duct on the left and into the lowest deep cervical node or upper thoracic node on the right.

Paratracheal nodes

The paratracheal nodes are also known as the recurrent laryngeal nodes as they accompany the recurrent laryngeal nerve. The majority of these nodes are found lateral to the trachea in the tracheo-oesophageal groove. Air in the trachea and oesophagus can create difficulties in assessing these lymph nodes.

They receive lymph from the larynx, piriform fossae, thyroid, oesophagus, trachea and pretracheal nodes, and drain into the thoracic duct on the left and the deep cervical chain on the right.

These nodes can lie posterior to the thyroid gland and may mimic parathyroid adenomata (Figure 4.14).

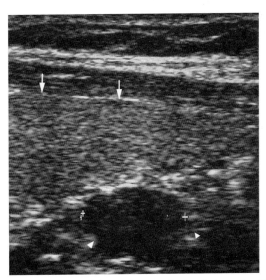

Figure 4.14 – Enlarged (10 mm) paratracheal node (arrowheads), posterior to the thyroid (arrowed), mimicking a parathyroid adenoma. Diagnosis: sarcoidosis.

They are distinguished from deep cervical nodes by the fact that they lie medial to the carotid artery and not lateral.

When this standard examination on both sides of the neck has been performed, the majority of the lymph node territories of the neck will have been covered. The lymph node territories that are not covered by this standard examination are now included for completeness.

Retropharyngeal nodes

These nodes cannot be assessed by ultrasound. They are often involved in nasopharyngeal and oropharyngeal primary tumours. This nodal area should always be included in the area scanned when the primary tumour is assessed by MRI or CT, thereby allowing a thorough assessment. There are two groups of nodes: the medial group lying near the midline in the retropharyngeal space, and the lateral nodes or nodes of Rouviere which lie just lateral to the longus colli muscle. The medial nodes are not normally seen whereas the nodes of Rouviere are well seen on MRI, particularly in younger patients.

Occipital nodes

At the very apex of the posterior triangle, sandwiched between the sternomastoid and trapezius muscles and the occipital bone superiorly, there exists a small cluster of nodes. They are usually involuted in adulthood but may be present in childhood. They drain chiefly into the spinal accessory chain and are difficult to identify with ultrasound.

Mastoid nodes

A small cluster of nodes exists just behind the ear, more numerous in the child than in the adult. These drain the auricle and external auditory meatus. Lymph then drains into the inferior parotid nodes and upper deep cervical nodes. In a co-operative child these nodes are readily identified but in the adult they have usually involuted. With the exception of melanoma they are rarely significant in the adult.

Ultrasound examination

Given the presence of so many lymph nodes in the 'normal' neck, how many lymph nodes should the operator expect to see on examining the neck with ultrasound? There are 300 lymph nodes in the neck (i.e. 150 on either side). A typical radical neck dissection should yield 30 nodes on careful pathological examination. So, how many lymph nodes should one expect to see with ultrasound? The answer is, 'It depends how hard you look!'. If you use a high frequency probe and spend hours examining all the lymph node territories you will find multiple nodes in all areas. But remember that finding benign innocent nodes is more difficult than detecting malignant lymph nodes. Pathological lymph nodes will leap out at you once you have mastered the basic ultrasound examination. Do not be worried if you cannot identify multiple nodes in all territories. Time spent looking for small insignificant nodes is time wasted. Once you have mastered the basic technique, a standard examination of the neck should take no more than 10–15 minutes. The greater the experience and the higher the frequency of probe used, the greater the number of lymph nodes that will be detected. Nodes involute as we become older. Lymph nodes are far more numerous in the younger individual; when scanning a 'normal' teenager's neck one would expect to detect 10–20 nodes with ease.

Classification systems

Just when we were getting to grips with the plethora of names and systems for the lymph nodes of the neck, the American Joint Committee on Cancer (AJCC) introduced the 'level terminology'.[3] The concept of 'levels' is driven by the fact that the extent and level of cervical node involvement is probably the most important prognostic factor for patients with a squamous cell primary. Node level is a highly significant predictor of survival. Stell,[4] in a review of 2058 patients with squamous cell carcinoma of the head and neck, showed that the 5-year survival rate for patients with nodes at level I (submandibular) was 34%, while it was only 4% for nodes at level IV (lower cervical).

It is important that we as radiologists embrace the concept of 'levels'. Surgeons base their treatment plan on the level of lymph node involvement, if any. The AJCC scheme aims to simplify the assessment of the neck, an aim which it mainly achieves. The levels scheme has evolved from Som's numeric nodal classification system,[5] but there are some important differences. Figure 4.15 is largely self-explanatory, but there are a few points worth highlighting:

1 Level I contains submental and submandibular nodes.

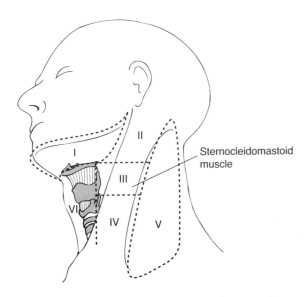

Figure 4.15 – The American Joint Committee on Cancer (AJCC) level classification.

2 Level V (the posterior triangle) is further subdivided into upper, middle and lower levels corresponding to the planes that divide II, III and IV (i.e. hyoid and cricothyroid membrane).
3 Retropharyngeal, parotid, mastoid and occipital nodes are not included in this level scheme.
4 Level V is defined as those nodes posterior to the posterior border of sternomastoid. Nodes deep to sternomastoid are therefore in II, III or IV.
5 Nodes of the upper spinal accessory chain may be included in the level II and III areas, in addition to the deep cervical chain.[6] Remember that superiorly the spinal accessory and deep cervical chains merge; differentiation between the two in the upper neck is academic.
6 Level VII nodes represent nodes in the superior mediastinum.
7 Classification systems for nasopharyngeal carcinoma and thyroid carcinoma differ.

The UICC–TNM classification[7] remains a largely anatomical classification. Care is needed, however, when using some of the terms employed in describing the lymph node groupings, e.g. dorsal cervical (superficial cervical) referring to the spinal accessory chain nodes.

Many other classification schemes exist[8] but, whatever system is used, it is important that surgeon and radiol-

ogist use the same terminology. Using a graphic format or standardised worksheet for recording lymph nodes is recommended. Recording the position and number of nodes on a standard diagram of the neck easily conveys the information the surgeon requires and eases comparison on follow-up studies. The standard examination described allows the ultrasound findings to be translated easily into readily identifiable territories for the surgeon. The surgeon or oncologist can easily translate that information into a level classification system.

Radiologists should not become too bogged down with classification systems. Use a system that allows for quick and efficient annotation of nodes detected.

Criteria of malignancy

There is no doubt that ultrasound is a sensitive examination for cervical lymphadenopathy.[9–14] Lymph nodes are easily detected once the operator is experienced in the ultrasound anatomy of the neck.

The problem then arises of trying to decide whether the lymph node detected is benign or malignant. Do criteria exist for differentiating between benign and malignant lymphadenopathy and, if so, are they valid? Such criteria do exist but while some are excellent in differentiation, others are poor. Commonly used criteria are:

1. Size

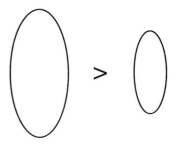

Figure 4.16 – Lymph node size as an indicator of malignancy.

The larger the lymph node detected, the greater the likelihood of malignancy; however nodes of up to 3–4 cm in length are often found in normal individuals, particularly children. Size alone is therefore a poor criterion for differentiating between benign and malignant lymph nodes. If a measurement is taken, then just as in CT[15] it is the axial or transverse diameter that has the best correlation with the increasing likelihood of metastatic disease. The selection of size as a criterion for differentiating between benign and malignant nodes must be based on compromise. A smaller transaxial diameter increases sensitivity, but with a subsequent decrease in specificity for detection of metastatic disease. Van den Brekel et al[10] analysed a range of minimal axial diameters in the N0 neck and found that a figure of 7 mm for submandibular and submental nodes, and 8 mm for all other nodes, gave an overall accuracy of 70%. This figure is lower than the transaxial diameters given in papers describing the use of CT for staging lymph node metastases (i.e. 10 mm and 11 mm).[15] An advantage of ultrasound over CT is that a transaxial diameter is a true axial or transverse diameter, i.e. it is taken at 90° to the longitudinal axis of the node. In the case of submandibular nodes, which are orientated in a relatively horizontal plane, diameters on CT are closer to being longitudinal measurements than true axial or transverse diameters.

Interestingly, Van den Brekel et al[9] state that the threshold for suspicion is much lower in patients where lymph node metastases are suspected (i.e. patients with a pre- or post-treatment known primary), and a minimal axial diameter of 4 mm is used for the selection of nodes for fine-needle aspiration cytology (FNAC).

In ultrasound the use of smaller axial diameters for suspicion of metastatic lymphadenopathy than those used in other imaging modalities results in a higher sensitivity but with a correspondingly lower specificity. This low specificity can be improved by ultrasound-guided FNAC. There is no doubt that size alone is a poor criterion, but axial diameters are helpful and can be used in conjunction with other criteria for differentiation. An increase in size on serial examination is a good sign of malignancy when searching for metastatic disease.

2. Shape

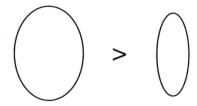

Figure 4.17 – Lymph node shape as an indicator of malignancy.

The shape of the lymph node is a far better indicator of benignity or malignancy than its size. Benign nodes tend to be elongated and fusiform in shape (Figure 4.18) whereas malignant nodes tend to have a greater transverse diameter, i.e. a more rounded shape. This was first hinted at by Sakai et al,[16] who stated that metastatic nodes show a more rounded configuration than non-metastatic nodes. Solbiati et al[17] first described the use of a long to short axis ratio (L/S ratio) in the distinction between benign (L/S > 2.0) and malignant nodes (L/S < 2.0). This was confirmed by Tohnosu and his colleagues,[18] who measured the short to long axis (S/L) ratio in cervical lymph nodes of patients with oesophageal cancer and compared this with the percentage cancer content on micro-analysis. An S/L ratio greater than 0.5 indicates a round node, whereas an S/L ratio of less than 0.5 indicates an oval, fusiform shaped node. The average cancer content in the metastatic lymph nodes with an S/L ratio under 0.5 was 26%, compared to 59% in nodes where the S/L ratio was greater than 0.5. Thus, the more rounded the node, the more likely it is to harbour metastatic disease. There is one exception to this rule: submandibular and submental nodes have a more ovoid and rounded outline than other cervical nodes,[19] and care therefore needs to be used when using shape as a criterion with nodes in the submental and submandibular regions.

A further study[14] has shown that an accuracy of 80% was achieved in an N0 population of patients with a primary tumour (92% sensitivity, 63% specificity) by using a ratio of more than 0.55 for the minimal/maximum transverse diameter, i.e. a rounded outline as the

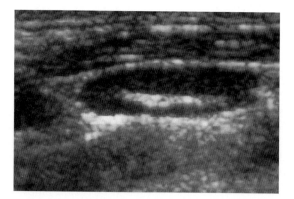

Figure 4.18 – Benign fusiform shaped lymph node with central echogenic hilus.

sole criterion. In this series the addition of other criteria did not improve accuracy.

3. Echogenic hilus

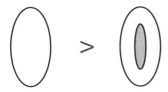

Figure 4.19 – Echogenic hilus as a criterion of malignancy.

A normal benign lymph node is an elliptical structure with an outer hypo-echoic cortex and a central bright echogenic hilus (Figure 4.20). A central echogenic line or hilus was first reported in 1985;[20] the echogenic structure was thought to represent fat within the node. Subsequent authors regarded the finding of this structure as a sign of benignity.[21, 22] Rubaltelli *et al*[23] were the first to correlate the sonographic and histological findings. They demonstrated that the central echogenic hilus is due to the parallel arrangement of the central lymphatic sinuses. This parallel arrangement serves as a series of specular reflectors which, when aligned parallel to the ultrasound beam, results in an echogenic hilus. Thus an echogenic hilus is a reflection of normal architecture within a lymph node; Rubaltelli and his colleagues therefore concluded that the finding of a central echogenic line is a valid criterion of benignity.

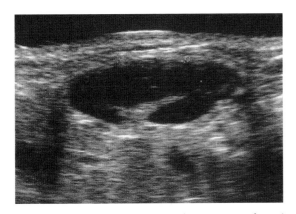

Figure 4.20 – Benign lymph node with prominent echogenic hilus continuous with surrounding fat.

While the echogenic hilus is an excellent sign of benignity, it is not foolproof. When a node undergoes malignant transformation there will be a point when only mild disruption of the central architecture has occurred, and remnants of the central hilus may be present in a node with metastatic deposits. This has been highlighted by Evans *et al*,[24] who demonstrated a central echogenic hilus in benign, lymphomatous (Figure 4.21), tuberculous and metastatic squamous cell carcinoma nodes.

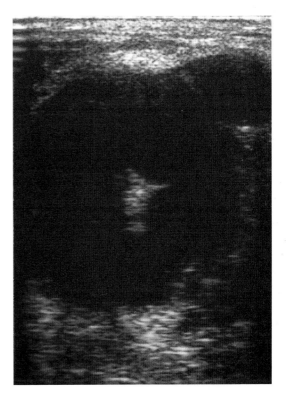

Figure 4.21 – Echogenic hilus in a rounded hypo-echoic node. Diagnosis: lymphoma.

Vassallo *et al*[25] have further analysed the hilus, assessing both the width of the hilus and the cortical width of the node. They conclude that a narrowed hilus in association with eccentric cortical widening should also be regarded as suspicious of malignancy (Figure 4.22). Thus a broad echogenic hilus is a good sign of benignity but not an absolute one. An absent hilus or a thin hilus with associated eccentric cortical widening should be regarded as an indicator of malignancy.

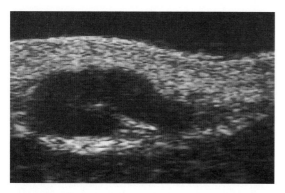

Figure 4.22 – Posterior triangle node. Eccentric cortical hypertrophy in association with a narrowed hilus.

4. Echogenicity

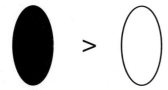

Figure 4.23 – Echogenicity as a criterion of malignancy.

Bruneton and Normand[26] first described the diffuse hypo-echogenicity of lymphomatous nodes, particularly non-Hodgkin's lymphoma. If a node has a fluid like appearance, i.e. is uniformly hypo-echoic with acoustic enhancement (pseudocystic appearance; Figure 4.24), then the features are suggestive of lymphoma. Others have also described this feature.[27] Bruneton and Normand[26] suggest that the appearances are due to the uniform cellularity of the node seen on histological examination.

Ahuja *et al*[28] showed that 90% of nodes involved in non-Hodgkin's lymphoma (NHL) in their series showed distal enhancement, compared to only 11% of nodes invaded by metastatic squamous cell carcinoma (cystic necrosis may account for this finding). Distal enhancement is therefore a significant and consistent differentiating feature between NHL and metastatic nodes. Metastatic nodes tend to have a heterogeneous appearance: the degree of overall hypo- or hyper-echogenicity does not correlate with the cancer content.

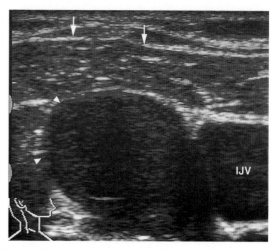

Figure 4.24 – Lower cervical node (arrowheads), deep to sternomastoid (arrowed). Diagnosis: lymphoma. High gain settings needed to demonstrate internal echoes. Note internal jugular vein (IJV).

5. Necrosis

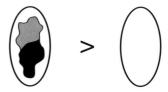

Figure 4.25 – Necrosis as a criterion of malignancy.

In a patient with a known primary the presence of necrosis in a node is a strong sign of malignancy. Necrosis may manifest itself as a true cystic area (Figure 4.26) within the node (cystic necrosis), or present as an area of hyperechogenicity within a node (coagulation necrosis). Coagulation necrosis is usually hyperechoic in relation to the cortex, but is not typically as echogenic as the surrounding fat and is not continuous with it (Figure 4.27). The central hilus is more echogenic than coagulation necrosis and is continuous with the surrounding fat. Coagulation necrosis typically occurs in metastases from keratinising squamous cell carcinoma. It may co-exist with areas of cystic necrosis in the same node; these tend to have a 'geographic' distribution within the node, predominantly central. The appearances are distinct from the central echogenic hilus and should not cause any diagnostic problem. Aspiration of these areas under ultrasound

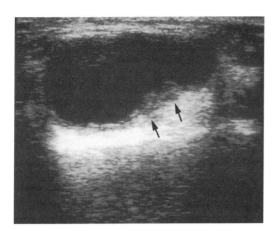

Figure 4.26 – Cystic necrosis in an intraparotid node. Note irregular thickening (arrowed) of capsule. Diagnosis: squamous cell carcinoma metastasis.

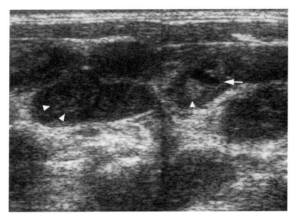

Figure 4.27 – Nasopharyngeal carcinoma metastases in posterior triangle. Note hyperechoic coagulation necrosis (arrowheads) in conjunction with areas of cystic necrosis (arrow).

control can sometimes yield fluid or pus-like material consistent with necrotic tumour. If the node contains a frankly necrotic area one should sample the more solid outer cortical area before aspirating the cystic medulla to improve the diagnostic yield.

Necrosis is often identified in tuberculous nodes, hence caution needs to be exercised when using this criterion. Tuberculous nodes tend to be clumped together with an associated inflamed surrounding interstitium.[29] Necrosis is common and the nodes may appear frankly malignant. The posterior triangle and supraclavicular regions are common sites for tuberculous nodes. Whenever cystic necrosis is detected in a

node, tuberculosis should always be considered in the differential diagnosis. Aspirates should be sent both for cytology and for microbiological culture.

6. Extracapsular spread

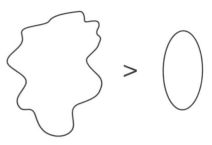

Figure 4.28 – Extracapsular spread as a criterion of malignancy.

Extracapsular spread can be detected by ultrasound. It implies a grave prognosis for the patient. The finding of extracapsular spread reduces the 2-year survival rate for the patient by 50%.[30]

The normal lymph node has a smooth margin. In malignant transformation the node has a rounded outline but tends to maintain a sharp border with the surrounding tissues. With advancing malignancy, the normal sharp smooth outline is lost (Figure 4.29) and extracapsular spread should be suspected. A spiculated margin or border should always be called extracapsular

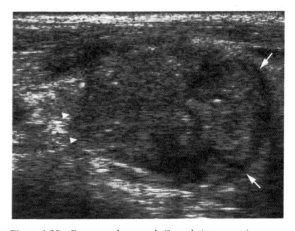

Figure 4.29 – Extracapsular spread. Coagulation necrosis present which has extended through the capsule (arrowheads). Note sharp border maintained laterally (arrows). Extracapsular spread confirmed at surgery.

spread. Invasion of adjacent muscle, salivary gland and vein from metastatic nodes have been identified (Figure 4.30); all are indicators of advanced extracapsular spread.

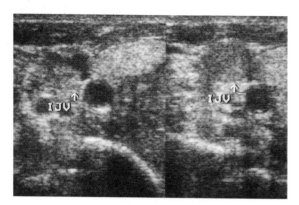

Figure 4.30 – Invasion of internal jugular vein (IJV) by metastatic squamous cell carcinoma nodes.

7. Colour flow

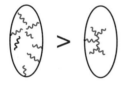

Figure 4.31 – Colour flow (vascular pattern) as a criterion of malignancy.

The superficial nature of cervical lymph nodes lends itself to assessment with high resolution colour Doppler and power Doppler imaging. Many centres[31-35] have attempted to differentiate between benign and malignant nodes using colour flow characteristics. Early studies[31,32] demonstrated flow in the hilum or centre of reactive lymph nodes. Others[36] showed that benign nodes are likely to have a central vascular pattern whereas a more disorganised peripheral vascular pattern is seen in malignant nodes. Histopathological studies[37,38] show that the main arteries and vein enter the node at the hilum, and spread in bundles of arteries and venules that course in alignment with the long axis of the lymph node. The cortex of the lymph node is fed by capillaries arising from these hilar and medullary vessels (Figure 4.1).

Tschammler *et al*[33] have further refined flow characteristics, stating that a benign node has a hilar vessel and/or a longitudinal vessel. Branches from this longitudinal vessel may be demonstrated. Malignant nodes may show the following changes:

- *displacement:* curved course of intranodal vessels

- *aberrant vessels:* characterised by one or more central vessel (no longitudinal vessel)

- *focal absence of perfusion*

- *subcapsular vessels* which do not originate from the hilar or longitudinal vessel.

When these criteria were used, Tschammler *et al* showed a 94% positive predictive value for malignancy when all four colour flow criteria were present but only a 67% positive predictive value if only one criterion was present. The loss of the echogenic hilus and a rounded outline were found to correlate well with the Doppler criteria for malignancy, the loss of normal architecture mirroring the abnormal vascular architecture in the malignant node (Figure 4.32).

Recent developments include the use of echo-contrast agents which allow improved delineation of blood flow distribution. Moritz *et al*[39] claim a 100% accuracy in differentiating between benign and malignant lymphadenopathy using ultrasound contrast media. Another interesting development is the use of 3D volumetric assessment of blood flow patterns in lymph nodes.[40] This will probably facilitate the detection of abnormal vasculature (especially subcapsular vessels) in lymph nodes. Abnormal tortuosity of intranodal vessels is also demonstrated with this technique and may

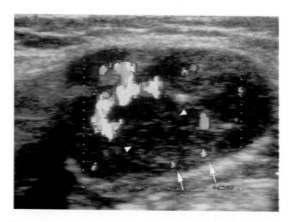

Figure 4.32 – Areas of focal absence of perfusion (arrowheads) and subcapsular vessels (arrows) on colour flow imaging.

prove to be another useful sign for the detection of malignancy (Figure 4.33). Remember that patterns of blood flow distribution are of more value than flow indices. Once colour flow gain settings are set correctly, the assessment of colour flow takes no more than the touch of a button and the positioning of a cursor. Flow pattern assessment should add no more than a few seconds to the examination of a particular node, provided the 'preset' has been entered correctly.

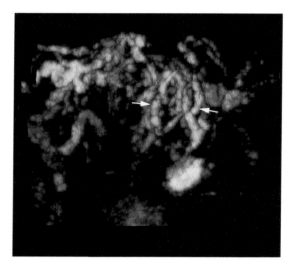

Figure 4.33 – 3D volumetric study. Note the tortuosity of the intranodal vessels (arrows).

8. Number

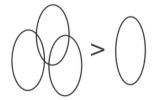

Figure 4.34 – Number of nodes as a criterion of malignancy.

The presence of a cluster of nodes in a draining region from a primary tumour would be regarded by some authors as a sign of malignancy.[9,10] If there are three or more borderline nodes in a particular region then they should be viewed with suspicion. Van den Brekel *et al*[9] state that these nodes should have a minimal axial diameter of not more than 2 mm less than the thresh-

old minimum axial measurement for that region (7 mm for submandibular and submental, 8 mm for subdigastric nodes).

There is no doubt that the presence of clusters of equivocal nodes in a particular region of the neck can be interpreted as a suspicious sign, however the finding of multiple small nodes in a region of the neck is not uncommon. Rouviere[2] states that in all areas of the neck the number of nodes found will be inversely proportional to their size. It is not uncommon to find six or seven small nodes in the submandibular region, and this finding alone should not be a cause for concern.

9. Calcification

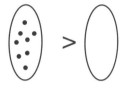

Figure 4.35 – Calcification as a criterion of malignancy.

Punctate areas of calcification (microcalcification) in a lymph node should immediately alert the radiologist to the possibility of a metastasis from a papillary carcinoma of the thyroid (Figure 4.36). Bright echogenic flecks can be made out in metastatic nodes[41] from papillary carcinoma of the thyroid. A diligent search of the thyroid for the primary should be carried out whenever such a sign is seen. FNAC of the lymph node

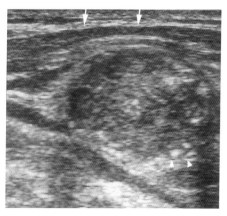

Figure 4.36 – Microcalcification (arrowheads) in a lower cervical node. The sternomastoid is arrowed. Diagnosis: metastatic papillary carcinoma.

should confirm the diagnosis. Occasionally metastases from a medullary cell carcinoma of the thyroid also display punctate echogenic foci.

Calcification is unlikely to be found in other metastatic nodes. Old tuberculous nodes are usually densely calcified and confusion should not occur.

Interpreting criteria of malignancy

How should we use these various proposed criteria? No single criterion is absolutely specific for benignity or malignancy, but shape, absence of hilus, irregular or spiculated outline, coagulation or cystic necrosis and disorganised peripheral colour flow pattern are all strong signs of malignancy. These signs should be used in summation – if a node displays several of these characteristics there is a high probability of malignancy.[42] Lymphoma should always be thought of in the differential diagnosis if rounded diffusely hypo-echoic nodes are detected.

The beauty of ultrasound is the ease with which ultrasound-guided FNA can be performed. Use the criteria to select the node for aspiration. Surgeons may not be impressed by an ultrasound report suggesting malignancy, but they will sit up and take notice when the accompanying supporting cytology report arrives! In our institution, the surgeons use the ultrasound report and cytology findings in combination when staging the neck. If the ultrasound report suggests malignancy but the FNAC is benign, the neck is still regarded as positive for malignancy and treatment planned accordingly. As in the management of breast cancer, the cytology and ultrasound findings are not viewed in isolation but in combination. Ultrasound in combination with FNAC is now our accepted method for staging the neck in patients with squamous cell carcinoma. In our hands sensitivity is 92%, specificity 83%, and the positive predictive value is 86% for the detection of metastatic nodes from squamous cell carcinoma.[43]

How does ultrasound in combination with FNAC compare with the other imaging modalities? In the only large series[44] that has compared all modalities – namely ultrasound (US), US-guided FNAC (USg FNAC), MRI and CT – ultrasound in combination with FNAC proved to be the most accurate technique. Accuracies of 86% (US), 100% (USg FNAC), 89% (CT) and 88% (MRI) were obtained. Far more significant, however, is the accuracy in necks where no nodes were palpable (N0 necks). This is the group of patients in whom the detection of lymph node metastases has a greater impact on management. Accuracy in the N0 group in Van den Brekel's study was 68% (US), 86% (USg FNAC), 66% (CT) and 75% (MRI).

It is in the assessment of this N0 group that radiologists can make the greatest impact. The number of patients who are under- or over-treated will be diminished if we can provide the surgeon with an accurate technique for evaluating the neck.

The lymphatics of the neck should no longer prove a daunting prospect for the radiologist. Ultrasound is now an excellent diagnostic tool, provided a simple methodical system is followed. Using the full range of criteria available, differentiation between reactive and malignant lymphadenopathy is now possible. In combination with FNAC, ultrasound is an accurate technique for evaluating the neck.

References

1. Herman PG, Lyonnet D, Fingerhut R, Tuttle RN. Regional blood flow to the lymph node during the immune response. *Lymphology* 1976; **9**: 101–104.

2. Rouviere H. *Anatomy Of The Human Lymphatic System.* Ann Arbor: Edward Brothers, 1938.

3. American Joint Committee on Cancer. *AJCC Cancer Staging Manual,* 5th edn. New York: Lippincott-Raven, 1997.

4. Stell PM, Morton RP, Singh SD. Cervical lymph node metastases: the significance of the level of the lymph node. *Clin Oncol* 1983; **9**: 101–107.

5. Som PM. Detection of metastasis in cervical lymph nodes: CT and MR criteria and differential diagnosis. *AJR* 1992; **158**: 981–969.

6. Byers RM, Weber RS, Andrews T, McGill D, Kare R, Wolf P. Frequency and therapeutic implications of 'skip metastases' in the neck from squamous cell carcinoma of the oral tongue. *Head & Neck* Jan 97: 14–19.

7. *UICC TNM Atlas,* 4th edn. Berlin: Springer Verlag, 1997.

8. Hajek PC, Salomonowitz E, Turk R, Tscholakoff D, Kumpan W, Czembirek H. Lymph nodes of the neck: evaluation with US. *Radiology* 1986; **158**: 739–742.

9. Van den Brekel M, Stel HV, Castelijns JA *et al.* Lymph node staging in patients with clinically negative examinations by ultrasound and ultrasound guided aspiration cytology. *Am J Surg* 1991; **162**: 362–366.

10. Van den Brekel M, Castelijns JA, Stel HV *et al.* Occult metastatic neck disease: detection with US and US guided fine needle aspiration cytology. *Radiology* 1991; **180**: 457–461.

11. Bruneton JN, Roux P, Caramella E, Demard F, Vallicioni J, Chauvel P. Ear, nose and throat cancer: ultrasound diagnosis of metastasis to cervical lymph nodes. *Radiology* 1987; **152**: 771–773.

12. Baatenburg de Jong RJ, Rongen RJ, Lameris JS, Harthoorn M, Verwoerd CDA, Knegt P. Metastatic neck disease: palpation vs ultrasound examination. *Arch Otolaryngol Head Neck Surg* 1989; **115:** 689–690.

13. Evans RM, Hodder S, Patton DW, Silvester KC. Lymph node metastases in patients with squamous cell carcinoma: utility of US and US-guided fine needle aspiration cytology. *Radiology* 1996; **201:** 412 (Abstract).

14. Takashima S, Sone S, Nomura N, Tomiyana N, Kobayashi T, Nakamura H. Non palpable lymph nodes of the neck: assessment with US and US guided fine needle aspiration biopsy. *J Clin Ultrasound* 1997; **25:** 283–292.

15. Van den Brekel M, Castelijns JA, Stel HV *et al*. Cervical lymph node metastasis: assessment of radiologic criteria. *Radiology* 1990; **177:** 379–384.

16. Sakai F, Kiyono K, Sone S *et al*. Ultrasonic evaluation of cervical metastatic lymphadenopathy. *J Ultrasound Med* 1988; **7:** 305–310.

17. Solbiati L, Rizzatto G, Bellotti E *et al*. High-resolution sonography of cervical lymph nodes in head and neck cancers: criteria for differentiation of reactive versus malignant nodes. *Radiology* 1988; **169**(P): 113 (Abstract).

18. Tohnosu N, Onoda S, Isono K. Ultrasonographic evaluation of cervical lymph node metastases in esophageal cancer with special reference to the relationship between the short to long axis ratio (S/L) and the cancer content. *J Clin Ultrasound* 1989; **17:** 101–106.

19. Ying M, Ahuja A, Brook F, Brown B, Metreweli C. Sonographic appearances and distribution of normal cervical lymph nodes in Chinese population. *J Ultrasound Med* 1996; **15:** 431–436.

20. Marchal G, Oyen R, Verschakelen J, Gelin J, Baert AL, Stessens RC. Sonographic appearances of normal lymph nodes. *J Ultrasound Med* 1985; **4:** 417–419.

21. Sutton RT, Reading CC, Charbonneau JW, James EM, Grant CS, Hay ID. Ultrasound guided biopsy of neck masses in post operative management of patients with thyroid cancer. *Radiology* 1988; **168:** 769–772.

22. Perin B, Gardellin G, Nisi E, Perini L, Lunghi F, Frasson P. Identificazione erografica di area iperecogena centrale nei linfondi. Segno di unfoademopatia benigna. *Radiol Med (Torino)* 1987; **74:** 535–538.

23. Rubaltelli L, Proto E, Salmaso R, Bortoletto P, Candiani F, Pierpaolo C. Sonography of abnormal lymph nodes in vitro: correlation of sonographic and histological findings. *AJR* 1990; **155:** 1241–1244.

24. Evans RM, Ahuja A, Metreweli C. The linear echogenic hilus in cervical lymphadenopathy – a sign of benignity or malignancy? *Clin Radiol* 1993; **47:** 262–264.

25. Vassallo P, Wernecke K, Roos N, Peters PE. Differentiation of benign from malignant superficial lymphadenopathy: the role of high resolution US. *Radiology* 1992; **183:** 215-220.

26. Bruneton JN, Normand F. Cervical lymph nodes. In: Bruneton JN, ed. *Ultrasonography of the Neck.* Berlin: Springer Verlag, 1987; pp 81–92.

27. Ishii JI, Fujii E, Suzuki H, Shinozuka K, Kawase N, Amagasa T. Ultrasonic diagnosis of oral and neck malignant lymphoma. *Bulletin of the Tokyo Medical and Dental University* 1992; **39:** 63–69.

28. Ahuja A, Ying M, Yang WT, Evans RM, King W, Metreweli C. The use of sonography in differentiating cervical lymphoma-tous nodes from cervical metastatic lymph nodes. *Clin Radiol* 1996; **51:** 186–190.

29. Ahuja A, Ying M, Evans RM, King W, Metreweli C. The application of ultrasound criteria for malignancy in differentiating tuberculous cervical adenitis from metastatic nasopharyngeal carcinoma. *Clin Radiol* 1995; **50:** 391–395.

30. Johnson JT. A surgeon looks at cervical lymph nodes. *Radiology* 1990; **175:** 607–610.

31. Turlington BS, Reading CC, Charboneau JW. Colour Doppler US in the neck: differentiating neoplastic from non-neoplastic lymphadenopathy. *Radiology* 1991; **181**(P): 177 (Abstract).

32. Ohnesorge I, Koenig H, Schill S, Wolf KJ. Colour coded duplex sonography of pathologically enlarged lymph nodes. *Radiology* 1991; **181**(P): 177 (Abstract).

33. Tschammler A, Ott G, Schant T, Seelbach-Goebel B, Schwager K, Hahn D. Lymphadenopathy: differentiation of benign from malignant disease – colour Doppler US assessment of intranodal angioarchitecture. *Radiology* 1998; **208:** 117–123.

34. Giovagnorio F, Caiazzo R, Avitto A. Evaluation of vascular patterns of cervical lymph nodes with power Doppler sonography. *J Clin Ultrasound* 1997; **25:** 71–76.

35. Chang DB, Yuan A, Yu CJ, Luh KT, Kuo HS, Yang PC. Differentiation of benign and malignant cervical lymph nodes with colour Doppler sonography. *AJR* 1994; **162:** 965–968.

36. Lencioni RA, Moretti M, Armillotta N, Bassi AM, Di Giuilio M, Bartolozzi C. Differentiation of benign and malignant superficial lymphadenopathy: value of high resolution power Doppler US. *Radiology* 1996; **201**(P): 225 (Abstract).

37. Semeraro D, Davies JD. The arterial blood supply of human inguinal lymph nodes. *J Anat* 1986; **144:** 221–233.

38. Gadre A, Briner W, O'Learly M. A scanning electron microscope study of the human cervical lymph node. *Acta Otolaryngol* 1994; **114:** 87–90.

39. Moritz JD, Ludwig AG, Kirchoff L, Volheim T, Oestmann JW. Contrast enhanced colour Doppler ultrasound in the evaluation of enlarged cervical lymph nodes in head and neck tumours. *Radiology* 1998; **209:** 310.

40. Metreweli C, Ahuja A. Work in progress: 3D colour power angio, does it have a potentially useful role in lymphadenopathy? *Eur J Ultrasound* 1998; **8,3:** S16–17 (Abstract).

41. Ahuja A, Chow L, Mok CO, King W, Metreweli C. Metastatic cervical lymph nodes in papillary carcinoma of the thyroid; ultrasound and histological correlation. *Clin Radiol* 1995; **50**(P): 391–395.

42. Evans RM, Ahuja A, Rhys Williams S, Waldron C, Van Hasselt CA, King W, Mcguire L. Ultrasound and ultrasound guided fine needle aspiration in cervical lymphadenopathy. *Br J Radiol* 1991; **64**(P): 58 (Abstract).

43. Hodder SC, Evans RM, Patton DW, Silvester KC. Prospective study of the use of ultrasound (in combination with Fine Needle Aspiration Cytology) in the staging of Neck Lymph Nodes in Oral Squamous Cell Carcinoma. *British Journal of Oral and Maxillofacial Surgery* (In press).

44. Van den Brekel MWM, Castelijns JA, Stel HV, Golding RP, Meyer CNL, Snow GB. Modern imaging techniques and ultrasound guided aspiration cytology for the assessment of neck node metastases: a prospective comparative study. *Eur Arch Otolaryngol* 1993; **250:** 11–17.

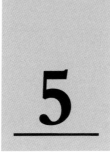

5

LUMPS AND BUMPS IN THE HEAD AND NECK

AT Ahuja

Introduction

Most textbooks discuss all lesions of the neck in terms of their frequency, but this chapter takes a different course in describing lesions according to their site (Figure 5.1). As described in Chapter 1, sonography of the neck should be carried out systematically, starting in the submental region and then proceeding to the different regions of the neck in sequential order. This protocol is important because it ensures that all the neck regions are scanned meticulously and the chance of missing a lesion is minimised. Also, as most lesions in the neck are site specific, their predetermined location in the neck, combined with ultrasound and clinical findings, provides a clue to the diagnosis.

We will therefore start with lesions in the submental area and proceed to discuss lesions in the other parts of the neck, following the scanning routine suggested earlier.

Masses in the submental region

The common masses in the submental region are:

Lymph nodes

A normal node or nodes are found in the submental area in the majority of individuals. These nodes are commonly oval, with an echogenic hilus.[1]

Metastatic nodes at this site are commonly from cancers of the tongue, anterior oral cavity, floor of the mouth, lip and anterior gingiva. However, one must note that in areas where nasopharyngeal carcinoma (NPC) is endemic, metastatic nodes in the submental area may be the only clue as to the presence of the primary. The submental region may also be the only site of recurrence in NPC patients who have been previously treated with radiotherapy.[2]

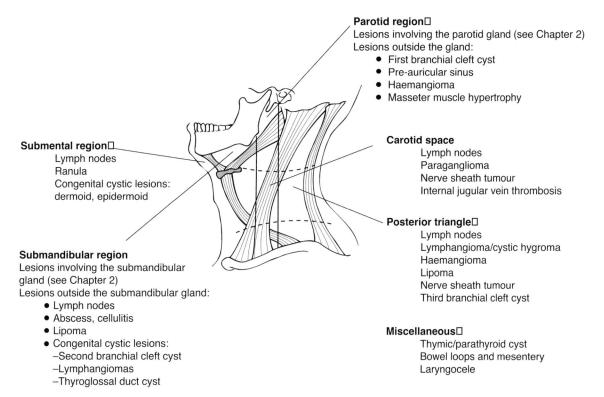

Parotid region
Lesions involving the parotid gland (see Chapter 2)
Lesions outside the gland:
- First branchial cleft cyst
- Pre-auricular sinus
- Haemangioma
- Masseter muscle hypertrophy

Submental region
Lymph nodes
Ranula
Congenital cystic lesions: dermoid, epidermoid

Carotid space
Lymph nodes
Paraganglioma
Nerve sheath tumour
Internal jugular vein thrombosis

Submandibular region
Lesions involving the submandibular gland (see Chapter 2)
Lesions outside the submandibular gland:
- Lymph nodes
- Abscess, cellulitis
- Lipoma
- Congenital cystic lesions:
  - Second branchial cleft cyst
  - Lymphangiomas
  - Thyroglossal duct cyst

Posterior triangle
Lymph nodes
Lymphangioma/cystic hygroma
Haemangioma
Lipoma
Nerve sheath tumour
Third branchial cleft cyst

Miscellaneous
Thymic/parathyroid cyst
Bowel loops and mesentery
Laryngocele

Figure 5.1 – Common masses in the neck.

Ranula

A ranula is a mucous retention cyst of the sublingual gland or, rarely, the minor salivary glands in the sublingual space. There are two forms:

1 *Simple ranula.* This is the most common form and invariably involves the sublingual gland. It remains in the floor of the mouth above the level of the mylohyoid. It is a true cyst, with an epithelial lining.
2 *Diving ranula.* When a simple ranula enlarges and ruptures into the submandibular space it forms a diving ranula which is really a pseudocyst and is not lined by epithelium.[3] It extends below the level of the mylohyoid.

ULTRASOUND APPEARANCES

A simple ranula is characteristically a unilocular, well-defined cystic lesion in the submental, sublingual space (Figure 5.2). It may contain fine internal echoes, usually debris.

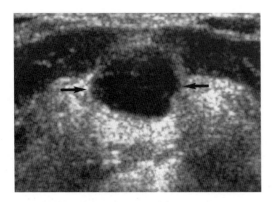

Figure 5.2 – Transverse sonogram of a cystic collection (arrows) restricted to the sublingual space. The appearances are those of a ranula. These are typically off midline in position, but may extend into the midline.

In a diving ranula the bulk of the cystic collection is in the submandibular space; a small beak is often seen within the sublingual space (Figure 5.3).

Congenital cystic lesions

Dermoid cysts are the rarest of the congenital cystic lesions in the neck. There are three different histological types:

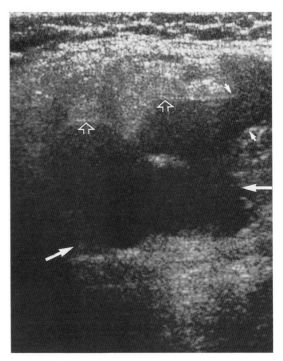

Figure 5.3 – Transverse sonogram of the submandibular space showing a heterogeneous collection (large arrows). Note its relationship to the submandibular gland (open arrows) and its extension into the sublingual space (small arrows). The appearances are typical of a diving ranula.

1 *Epidermoid or epidermal cyst.* This is the dermoid most commonly found in the head and neck. It is surrounded by a fibrous capsule and has an epithelial lining. It does not contain skin appendages.
2 *Dermoid.* This also has an epithelial lining and contains skin appendages.
3 *Teratoid cyst.* This is histologically similar to the epidermoid but contains connective tissue elements.[4] It is the least commonly encountered dermoid.

Only 7% of all dermoids occur in the head and neck. They are located in or slightly off the midline.

ULTRASOUND APPEARANCES

An epidermoid is usually well defined; although cystic, it exhibits a pseudo-solid appearance on ultrasound with uniform internal echoes (Figure 5.4). In congenital cysts this appearance is thought to be caused by cellular material within the cyst.[5]

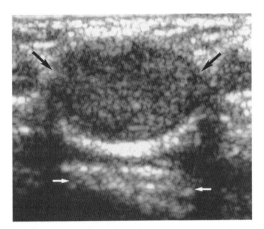

Figure 5.4 – Transverse sonogram showing a pseudo-solid appearance of an epidermoid cyst (black arrows). Note the homogeneous internal architecture suggesting a solid consistency. However the posterior enhancement is a clue to the cystic nature of the lesion (arrows).

Dermoids have mixed internal echoes because of their fat content (Figure 5.5) and may show the presence of osseo-dental structures within, seen as echogenic foci with dense shadowing.

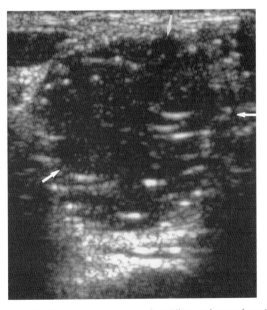

Figure 5.5 – Transverse sonogram of a midline, submental cystic mass with heterogeneous internal echoes (arrows). The location and ultrasound appearances suggest a dermoid.

In the absence of demonstrable fat and osseo-dental structures on ultrasound, one cannot differentiate between a dermoid and an epidermoid.

Masses in the submandibular region

Lesions in the submandibular space can be subdivided into those that involve the submandibular salivary gland and those that are outside the gland.

The role of ultrasound as the initial investigation of choice in evaluating the submandibular gland is well established.[6-8] The sonologist must be alert to the fact that a pedunculated mass arising from the apex of the superficial lobe of the parotid gland may encroach on the submandibular space and be mistaken for a submandibular mass. If the lesion is not recognised as parotid in origin by both the clinician and the sonologist, a submandibular approach will be made to this parotid lesion, resulting in poor surgical control of the facial nerve.[9]

The common extraglandular lesions are:

Lymph nodes

Most individuals have demonstrable nodes in the submandibular area. Malignant nodes at this site are commonly: lymphoma[10,11] and metastatic nodes from cancers of the tongue, anterior oral cavity, floor of the mouth, lip and anterior gingiva. In orientals, enlarged intraparotid nodes and nodes in the submandibular region, with or without salivary gland masses, should alert the sonologist to the possibility of Kimura's disease.[12]

Abscess, cellulitis

In the antibiotic era, the incidence of cervical abscess and cellulitis is low. It is commonly seen in postoperative patients, drug users and immunocompromised patients. Abscess and cellulitis in the submandibular area originate from suppurative adenopathy, salivary gland infection, dental abscess or mandibular osteomyelitis, or following radiotherapy to the area.

Prior to aspiration or surgery it is important to delineate the abscess and its anatomical relations. In addition, one can identify complications of an abscess such as a venous thrombosis or carotid involvement. The sonologist must always identify the entire extent of the abscess, particularly its lower limit.

ULTRASOUND APPEARANCES

In cellulitis there is no fluid collection and the area shows a diffuse reticulated (cobblestone; Figure 5.6), hyperechoic appearance with hypo-echoic septa.

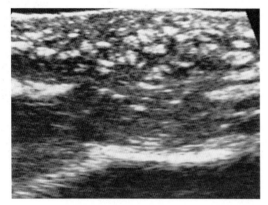

Figure 5.6 – Transverse sonogram of the submandibular region showing a cobblestone reticulated appearance. The appearances are typical of cellulitis, commonly post radiotherapy.

An abscess is seen as an ill-defined, irregular collection with thick walls and internal debris (Figure 5.7). It may be unilocular or multilocular, with oedema of adjacent soft tissues. There is loss of the fascial planes and the presence of adjacent inflammatory nodes. The rim of the abscess may demonstrate hypervascularity on colour flow imaging.

The differential diagnosis must always include a necrotic malignant node with superadded infection. Such nodes also have thick, irregular walls with internal debris and may show a rim of vascularity. Fine-needle aspiration (FNAC) will distinguish between the two.

Lipoma

Lipomas are benign encapsulated lesions which are typically subcutaneous or submucosal in location. They tend to displace rather than infiltrate adjacent structures. About 13% of all lipomas occur in the head and neck. In females they are typically located adjacent to the clavicle, whereas in men they are located in the posterior triangle. Infiltrating lipomas are rare in the

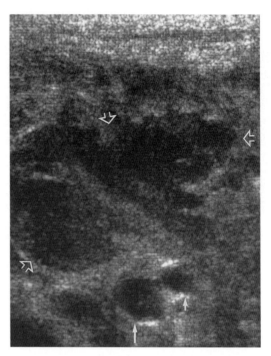

Figure 5.7 – Transverse sonogram showing an ill-defined, heterogeneous collection (open arrows) anterior to the common carotid artery (small arrow) and the internal jugular vein (large arrow). The appearances are those of an abscess.

head and neck. Following surgery the recurrence rate is high (50%), probably due to microscopic infiltration of adjacent soft tissues. The recurrence rate for infiltrating lipomas is even higher – 62.5%.[13]

Lipomas have typical sonographic features, these ease their identification.[14]

ULTRASOUND APPEARANCES

Head and neck lipomas (Figure 5.8):

- are compressible, well-defined, elliptical masses parallel to the skin surface
- are hyperechoic relative to the adjacent muscle with heterogeneous internal echoes
- contain linear echogenic lines at right angles to the ultrasound beam
- display no distal enhancement or attenuation
- do not demonstrate significant vascularity within or around the mass.

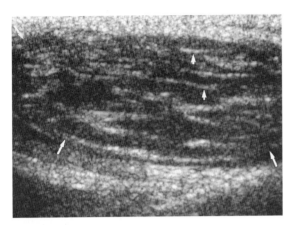

Figure 5.8 – Transverse sonogram of a well-defined mass (large arrows) with linear streaks parallel to the skin surface (small arrows). The appearances are those of a lipoma.

Congenital cystic lesions

BRANCHIAL CLEFT CYST (BCC)

Of all the branchial cleft anomalies, 95% arise from the remnants of the second branchial apparatus. The most common form of this lesion is a cystic mass without a sinus or fistula at the angle of the mandible.[9] Second BCCs are more common in children and young adults.[9,15] 97% of BCC linings contain lymphoid tissue (either nodular or diffuse) which can hypertrophy during an infection; BCCs therefore often present following an upper respiratory tract infection.[16] The site of the BCC is embryologically defined in the posterior sub-mandibular region at the angle of the mandible. Typically, a second BCC is located superficial to the common carotid artery (CCA) and internal jugular vein (IJV), posterior to the submandibular gland and along the medial and anterior margin of the sternocleidomastoid muscle, commonly near the level of the angle of the mandible. A second BCC may occasionally be associated with a sinus or fistula that opens into the tonsillar fossa. The tract descends along the anterior border of the sternocleidomastoid muscle and may open on to the skin surface anywhere along this path.

Ultrasound appearances

Uninfected branchial cysts. Most of the branchial cysts demonstrate the typical appearances of a cyst in that they are well defined and anechoic with no internal debris and show posterior enhancement (Figure 5.9).[17,18] However, some cysts may exhibit a pseudo-

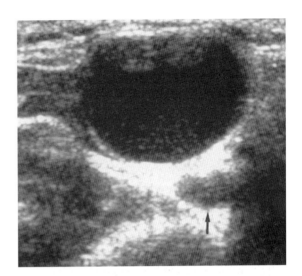

Figure 5.9 – Longitudinal sonogram of an uninfected, predominantly anechoic branchial cyst with thin walls, with posterior enhancement. Faint internal debris and anterior reverberation artefact are seen within the cyst. Note its relationship to the carotid artery (black arrow).

solid appearance with uniform internal echoes (Figure 5.10). This is probably due to the presence of variable quantities of mucus, cholesterol crystals, debris, lymphocytes and epithelial cells within the cyst.[5,18]

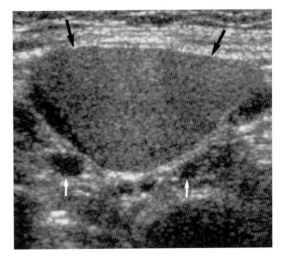

Figure 5.10 – Transverse sonogram of a branchial cyst showing a pseudo-solid appearance (black arrows), anterior to the carotid bifurcation (white arrows). On compression swirling echoes will be seen within the cyst.

Infected branchial cysts. These cysts are usually ill defined and thick walled; they contain internal debris and septa (Figure 5.11). The appearances are secondary to repeated infection or haemorrhage. The sonologist must be aware of the fact that cystic metastases from a papillary carcinoma may have a similar appearance.[19] A detailed examination of the thyroid and FNA of the cystic lesion must therefore be performed.

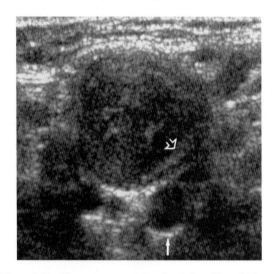

Figure 5.11 – Transverse sonogram of an infected branchial cyst with thick walls (open arrow) and internal debris. Note the position of the cyst in close proximity to the carotid artery (arrow).

In the case of branchial cysts, the operator must be aware that they may have cranial, parapharyngeal (between carotid artery and lateral pharyngeal wall) extensions which may not always be depicted on ultrasound. A CT or MR scan is therefore indicated in cases where the extent of the lesion cannot be identified by ultrasound.

LYMPHATIC MALFORMATIONS

Lymphatic malformations are congenital abnormalities that arise when developing lymphatics fail to establish communication with developing veins.[20,21] They can be divided into three types:
1 *cystic hygromas:* lymphatic malformations with large lymphatic spaces
2 *cavernous lymphangiomas:* these have smaller spaces and develop from buds that would have formed terminal lymphatics[21]

3 *capillary* or *simplex lymphangiomas:* these contain the smallest spaces.

The greatest lymphatic development occurs early in childhood, the majority of these lesions present in patients under two years of age. Solitary cystic hygromas may be seen in young adults in the submandibular region and the posterior triangle. It is believed that these are usually post-traumatic rather than congenital in origin.[16]

Large cystic hygromas are the type most commonly seen; the remainder of the discussion therefore focuses on the clinical manifestations and ultrasound appearances of cystic hygroma. 50–60% present at birth, another 30% presenting by 2 years of age.[15] In an infant they are commonly located in the *posterior triangle* and the cervicothoracic junction, whereas in adults they are seen in the submental, submandibular and parotid space. They present clinically as painless compressible masses and, when sufficiently large, transilluminate. Following haemorrhage, however, they can become rigid, suddenly increasing in size to compress adjacent structures and cause pain and facial paralysis.[16]

The primary role of imaging is to demonstrate the anatomic extent of the hygroma before surgery. This is easier said than done, as cystic hygromas are trans-spatial (involving more than one anatomical space) and insinuate themselves between the major neurovascular structures in the neck. Particular attention must be paid to the inferior extent as 10% may extend into the mediastinum.[22] Although ultrasound can make the initial diagnosis of cystic hygroma, CT or MR imaging is necessary to map the full extent of large lesions.

Ultrasound features

- Small lesions may be unilocular but larger ones are multilocular.

- Extensive vascularity may be seen within the septa.

- Cystic hygromas are trans-spatial and follow no obvious anatomic boundaries, extending into multiple cervical spaces.

Uninfected lesions are seen as multiple, compressible cysts of varying sizes with thin walls and intervening septa (Figures 5.12, 5.13) which infiltrate between and around neurovascular structures. Although they may be large in size they do not cause mass effect or displacement of adjacent structures. In fact, adjacent muscles and vessels cause indentations on the hygroma.

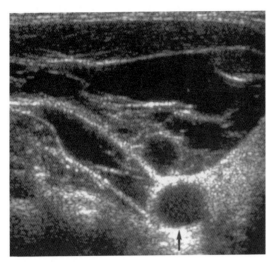

Figure 5.12 – Transverse sonogram of a cystic hygroma showing multiple cystic spaces and septa. Note its relationship to the common carotid artery (arrow).

In *infected* or *haemorrhagic lesions* the cyst walls are irregular, contain internal debris, are incompressible and mimic a solid lesion. They may produce a mass effect and compress the trachea, causing respiratory distress.[23]

THYROGLOSSAL DUCT CYST (TDC)

A thyroglossal duct cyst is a congenital anomaly related to the thyroglossal duct. It is thought to represent segments of the duct that fail to regress and consequently differentiate into epithelial-lined cysts,[24] developing anywhere along the course of the duct remnant.[25] The majority are related to the hyoid bone. About 25–65% occur in the infrahyoid neck, 15–50% occur at the level of the hyoid, and 20–25% are suprahyoid in location encroaching upon the submental region. TDCs occurring above the thyroid cartilage are usually midline whereas those at the level of the cartilage are off midline.

Patients usually present with a painless midline mass and there is often a history of previous incision and drainage at the site. About 50% present before the age of 10 years, the second group of patients presenting in young adulthood.

TDCs are diagnosed clinically and the role of imaging is to confirm the clinical diagnosis and provide preoperative information regarding the presence of a solid component within the cyst. Ultrasound is ideally suited to provide this information and in most cases no other imaging is necessary.

Ultrasound features

The typical ultrasound appearance of a TDC has been described as that of an anechoic, well-circumscribed cyst with increased through transmission.[23,26,27] In our experience, however, this is not the case. We have found four patterns:[28]

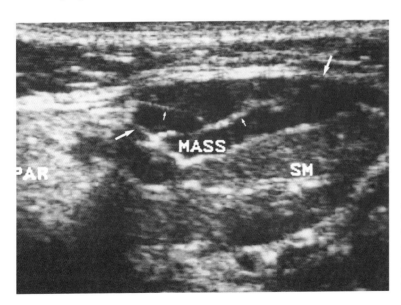

Figure 5.13 – Transverse sonogram of a cystic hygroma (mass, large arrows) showing a cystic lesion with septa (small arrows) in close proximity to the submandibular gland (SM) and parotid gland (PAR). At this site, lymphangiomas in adults are said to be post-traumatic in origin.

1 anechoic – 27.5% (probably representing unin-fected TDCs; Figure 5.14)
2 hypo-echoic with internal debris – 17.5%
3 heterogeneous pattern – 27.5% (probably due to repeated infections, haemorrhage due to previous aspirations; Figure 5.15)
4 uniformly echogenic pseudo-solid appear-ance – 27.5% (probably due to the proteinaceous content of the cyst thought to be secreted by the epithelial lining; Figure 5.16).[25]

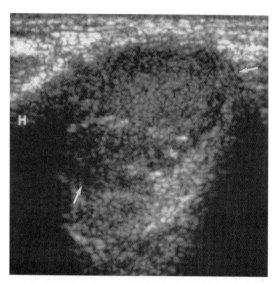

Figure 5.16 – Longitudinal sonogram of an infrahyoid thyroglos-sal duct cyst (arrows) showing a pseudo-solid appearance. Note that it is just below the level of the hyoid bone (H).

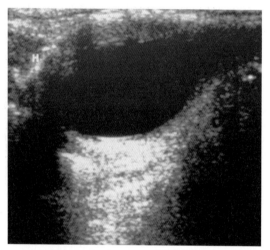

Figure 5.14 – Longitudinal sonogram of an uninfected, infrahy-oid thyroglossal duct cyst. Note the anechoic nature of the cyst and posterior enhancement. The hyoid is identified as 'H'.

Ultrasound also identifies the presence of any solid component within the cyst; malignant degeneration of the epithelial lining of a TDC, although rare, has been reported.[29,30] Ultrasound-guided fine-needle aspiration cytology (FNAC) is therefore recom-mended in any case of a solid component within a TDC.

Although ultrasound does not identify the tract in all cases, it is not critical because, irrespective of the site, size and appearance of a TDC, a Sistrunk procedure is recommended.[31] This entails resection of the cyst and any remaining tract, together with excision of the middle third of the hyoid bone. Incomplete resection invariably results in recur-rence.

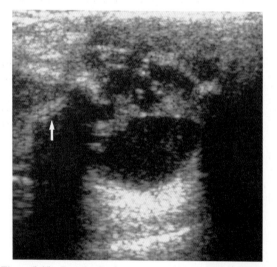

Figure 5.15 – Longitudinal sonogram of an infected thyroglossal duct cyst with internal debris and septa. The hyoid is identified by an arrow.

Masses in the parotid region

Lesions in the parotid region can be divided into those involving the parotid gland and those that are extra-glandular. The role of ultrasound in evaluating the parotid gland is well documented[8,32,33] and has been dis-cussed in Chapter 2.

The common extraglandular lesions are:

Masseter muscle hypertrophy (MMH)

Masseter muscle hypertrophy may be unilateral or bilateral. The aetiology is obscure, but most patients have habitual clenching or grinding habit of the jaw, especially during sleep. The highest incidence is in the second and third decades of life and there is no sex predilection.

Treatment, if indicated, consists of masseteric resection and reduction of associated bony hyperostosis. However, many surgeons are hesitant to recommend surgery for this benign condition, particularly as there is an associated risk of facial nerve damage and considerable postoperative morbidity. The known actions of botulinum toxin appear to offer potential benefit to patients that require treatment and in some centres this is now the primary form of treatment. Following injection of botulinum toxin, it is not possible for the patient to clench the teeth firmly due to functional denervation of the jaw; it is postulated that this period of forced inactivity is sufficient to break the habit of clenching/grinding.[34]

Ultrasound has a role to play in patients with MMH as it can eliminate other causes of focal swelling and evaluate and compare muscle size. The toxin can be injected under ultrasound control. Ultrasound is also useful in monitoring the size of the muscle after treatment.

First branchial cleft cyst

A first BCC arises from abnormal embryogenesis of the first branchial apparatus and accounts for 8% of all branchial cleft abnormalities. It may be associated with bony changes in the form of a tract through the external auditory canal and temporal bone.[35] These cysts occur in and around the parotid gland, external auditory canal and the angle of the mandible. The typical patient with a first BCC is a middle-aged woman with a history of multiple parotid abscesses unresponsive to antibiotics and drainage. There may be associated otorrhoea. The sonologist may be the first person to suggest the diagnosis.

ULTRASOUND FEATURES

- The cyst may be located within the parotid gland or just adjacent to it. It may be mistaken for a parotid cyst.

- Although the ultrasound appearances are similar to those of a second BCC, in our experience the most common is a pseudo-solid appearance with uniform internal echoes and posterior enhancement (Figure 5.17). Infected cysts with heterogeneous internal echoes are frequently mistaken for the more common Warthin's tumour, particularly in males.

- If the cyst is infected, enlarged inflammatory intraparotid nodes are seen.

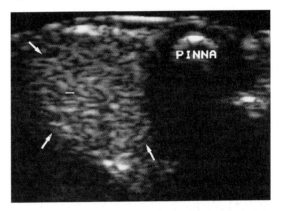

Figure 5.17 – Transverse sonogram showing an echogenic cyst (arrows) closely related to the pinna. The location and appearance are suggestive of a first branchial cleft cyst.

Although the diagnosis is made on ultrasound, CT is necessary to evaluate any associated bony abnormality.

Pre-auricular sinus

Pre-auricular sinuses are the most common congenital abnormality in the head and neck. They result from the entrapment of ectodermal epithelium in the first branchial arch elements of the external ear.[36] They do not involve branches of the facial nerve. While most remain asymptomatic, a small minority become infected and this may cause chronic discharge, repeated abscess formation and scarring. Sonography can detect pre-auricular sinuses and their branching pattern, providing the surgeon with valuable pre-operative information.

ULTRASOUND FEATURES

- The sinus may be branching or non-branching (Figure 5.18a).

95

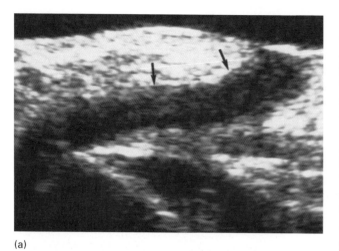

(a)

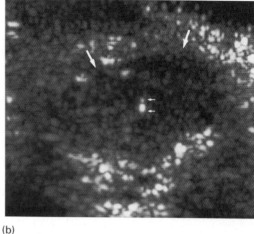

(b)

Figure 5.18 – Longitudinal sonogram in the pre-auricular region showing (a) a non-branching sinus (arrows). (b) Note the associated collection (large arrows) and gas within (small arrows).

- There is a pseudo-glandular component associated with the sinus, due to accumulation of secretions (Figure 5.18b). On ultrasound it is frequently well defined and globular, showing uniform internal echoes.

- The width of the sinus is usually 3–4 mm.

- Ultrasound accurately identifies the relationships of the sinus to the anterior crux of the helix, the groove between the helix and the tragus, and the superficial temporal artery.

- Gas may be seen within the sinus and its ramifications.

Haemangiomas

They are common in the trunk and the extremities but uncommon in the head and neck region (approximately 15% of haemangiomas).[37,38] The masseter muscle is the most common site (36%), followed by trapezius muscle (24%), sternomastoid (10%), periorbital muscles (10%) and temporalis muscle (8%).[38,39] Vascular malformations may have large (cavernous) spaces, capillary elements, lymphatic elements or combinations of these.[21,40]

The role of imaging is to identify the exact anatomic location and the extent of the mass before therapy. Large haemangiomas may be trans-spatial. The diagnosis is readily made by ultrasound, particularly when the presence of a phlebolith is demonstrated, but MRI best depicts the exact anatomic location and extent of the lesion.

ULTRASOUND FEATURES[41,42]

- Haemangiomas are hypo-echoic.

- They have a heterogeneous echopattern.

- Multiple sinusoidal spaces are seen within the mass (Figure 5.19).

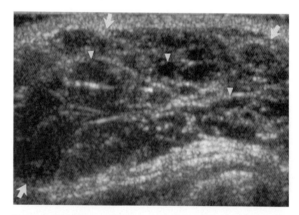

Figure 5.19 – Transverse sonogram of a haemangioma, showing a hypo-echoic mass (arrows) with multiple vascular spaces within (arrowheads). On real-time scanning one will often see slow flow within these spaces. Colour Doppler may also demonstrate sluggish flow.

- Colour flow imaging can demonstrate the presence of slow flow. However, this is not a consistent feature.

- Phleboliths are seen in about 20% of cases (Figure 5.20). However, our recent experience shows that one can identify the presence of a phlebolith in almost 60% of cases when a careful search is made.

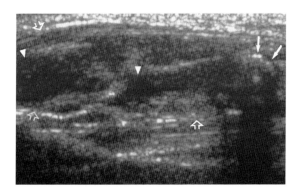

Figure 5.20 – Longitudinal sonogram of a haemangioma, showing a hypo-echoic mass (open arrows) with vascular spaces (arrowheads). The presence of a phlebolith (arrows) confirms the diagnosis.

Masses along the carotid artery and internal jugular vein

The 'carotid space' contains nerves, vessels and nodes. The most common lesions at this site are therefore related to these structures.

Paraganglioma

Paragangliomas, also known as glomus tumours, arise from neural crest cells within the vessel wall. Almost all the paragangliomas in the head and neck region occur:
1 in the carotid body at the carotid bifurcation – carotid body tumours (CBT)
2 along the nodose ganglion of the vagus nerve – glomus vagale
3 along the jugular ganglion of the vagus nerve – glomus jugulare
4 around the Arnold and Jacobson nerves in the middle ear – site of the glomus tympanicum.

Ultrasound can only evaluate the carotid body tumour, and so the rest of this discussion will focus on it. CBTs present as pulsatile, painless masses in the anterior tri-

angle just below the angle of the mandible. They are slightly more common in women than men, and may be bilateral or associated with other head and neck paragangliomas. In patients with a family history of paragangliomas the prevalence rate of such multiple tumours is 25–33%.[43–45] The key to the identification of a CBT is its location at the carotid bifurcation, straddling the bifurcation and splaying the vessels.

ULTRASOUND FEATURES

- The characteristic location of the tumour at the carotid bifurcation is the first clue.

- Colour flow imaging demonstrates the encasement of the bifurcation by tumour particularly well (Figure 5.21). It also shows the vascularity within the tumour (ranging from hypovascular to hypervascular).

- The tumour is frequently well defined.

- CBT is hypo-echoic relative to adjacent structures, solid and non-calcified.

- Always evaluate the other side as these tumours may be bilateral.

When the bifurcation is seen within the tumour, the diagnosis can be made with confidence. In some instances, however, the mass displaces and splays the

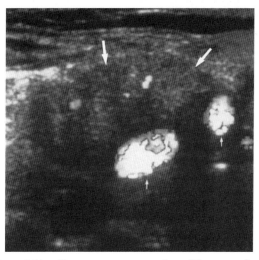

Figure 5.21 – Transverse sonogram of a solid tumour (large arrows) encasing the bifurcation of the common carotid artery (small arrows). The location of the vessels within the tumour is characteristic of a carotid body tumour.

vessels without encircling them and may demonstrate only minimal vascularity. In these cases the diagnosis is difficult and differential diagnosis includes malignant nodes or nerve sheath tumours (Figure 5.22).

Although ultrasound readily makes the diagnosis, MRI or CT is indicated to rule out the presence of other head and neck paragangliomas (particularly in patients with a family history).[15]

Nerve sheath tumours

Schwannomas and neurofibromas are the nerve sheath tumours most commonly found in the head and neck. Neurofibromas are unencapsulated tumours of the axons and Schwann cells, infiltrating and enlarging the nerves. They are frequently multiple and associated with neurofibromatosis type 1. Malignant change is far more likely in the setting of neurofibromatosis than it is for a solitary tumour.[46] Schwannomas contain Schwann cells but no other neural elements.[47] They are encapsulated and well circumscribed.

The common sites in the neck include the vagus nerve, ventral and dorsal cervical nerve roots, the cervical sympathetic chain, and the brachial plexus. The location of these tumours is the most important clue to

their origin, i.e. tumours from the vagus nerve will be seen in the anterior triangle, tumours from the cervical nerve roots in the posterior triangle, and those from the sympathetic chain are closely related to the longus colli muscle. FNA of these tumours may trigger excruciating pain (considered diagnostic)[48] and it is important to recognise these lesions before biopsy.

ULTRASOUND FEATURES

- Both schwannomas and neurofibromas show a hypo-echoic, heterogeneous echopattern.[49]

- A pseudocystic appearance with posterior enhancement is commonly seen with both tumours[50,51] and this may lead to confusion. Neurofibromas, however, do not always show this posterior enhancement.[52]

- Neurofibromas may be lobulated, and schwannomas may show a true well-defined cystic component within the tumour (Figure 5.23).[48]

- The contours of the tumour are well defined; irregular borders may suggest malignant change.[52]

- The nerve immediately adjacent to the tumour may be thickened, producing a tapering appearance to

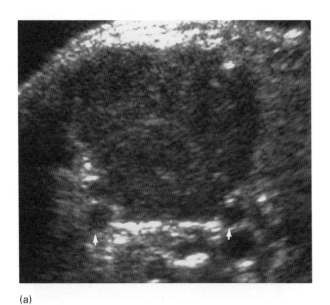
(a)

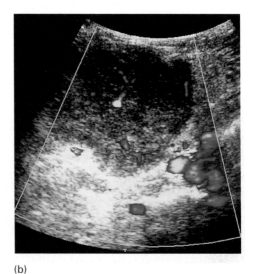
(b)

Figure 5.22 – Transverse sonogram of a large, ill-defined, hypo-echoic mass splaying the carotid bifurcation (a). Although its position is consistent with a carotid body tumour, it is relatively hypovascular (b). At surgery it was found to be a malignant node with extra-capsular spread. The encasement of the bifurcation within the mass is a more reliable sign of a carotid body tumour.

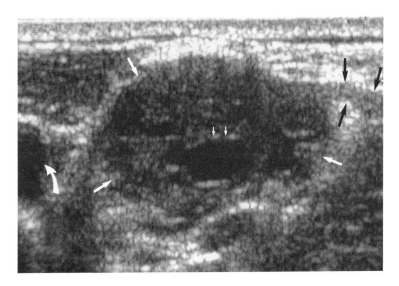

Figure 5.23 – Transverse sonogram of a hypo-echoic mass (white arrows) with adjacent exiting/entering nerve (black arrows) consistent with a nerve sheath tumour. Note the small, well-defined cystic area within the tumour (small arrows). Curved arrow identifies the common carotid artery.

the oval tumours. The presence of nerve thickening is the best clue to the nature of these tumours (Figure 5.24).[49]

● Histologically, schwannomas are more vascular than neurofibromas. Colour flow imaging also demonstrates this increased vascularity,[49] which is extremely sensitive to pressure. Even mild transducer pressure obliterates intratumoural vascularity.

Despite the histological differences between schwannomas and neurofibromas, the sonographic features have not allowed reliable distinction between the two.

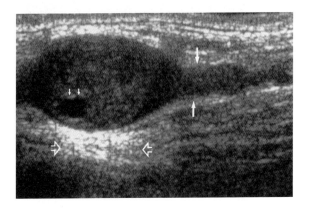

Figure 5.24 – Longitudinal sonogram of a nerve sheath tumour with adjacent thickened nerve (large arrows), cystic space within the tumour (small arrows) and posterior enhancement (open arrows).

These lesions are commonly mistaken for lymph nodes. Normal lymph nodes along the cervical chain are hypo-echoic and oval in shape, with sharp borders and a normal hilar structure within.[1] Normal nodes also do not show posterior enhancement. Differentiating nerve sheath tumours from malignant nodes is more difficult as these nodes are round, hypo-echoic, often do not demonstrate the hilum and may have areas of internal cystic necrosis. Lymphomatous nodes also show frequent (95%) posterior enhancement.[11]

Vascular lesions

The role of ultrasound in examination of the head and neck vessels is discussed in Chapter 9. We will confine our discussion to jugular vein thrombosis.

Jugular vein thrombosis

The right internal jugular vein is normally larger than the left, presumably reflecting the dominant right-sided drainage of the cerebral veins.

The causes of internal jugular vein thrombosis include: placement of a central venous line, trauma, surgery, infection, neoplasm and intravenous drug abuse. The clinical presentation depends on the phase of the thrombosis. In the acute thrombophlebitic phase it mimics infection, the patient presenting with fever and a warm tender neck swelling. In the chronic phase, the patient may present with a painless, hard mass mimicking a tumour.

Ultrasound appearances

Acute phase:

- There is absence of fascial planes between the IJV and adjacent soft tissues, with associated cellulitis.

- The thrombus is seen as an echogenic structure within the IJV and may cause venous distension. The presence of the thrombus may be a subtle feature and be better seen on a Valsalva manoeuvre. Lack of compressibility may also help.

- On colour flow imaging no flow is seen in an echogenic venous thrombus, whereas tumour thrombus within the IJV shows vascularity within the thrombus (Figure 5.25).

Chronic phase:

- The fascial planes around the vessel are preserved and there is no evidence of cellulitis.

- The thrombus is well organised and echogenic.

Abnormalities in the IJV are often overlooked as many sonologists do not pay as much attention to the IJV as to the CCA. The other reason is that the IJV may be collapsed and is therefore not identified. Internal jugular vein thrombosis is frequently misdiagnosed as an abnormal lymph node, which is a more common abnormality. Sluggish venous flow may cause internal echoes within the IJV and be mistaken for a thrombus. This is a common cause of false positive results.

It is therefore essential to evaluate the IJV carefully, if necessary with a Valsalva manoeuvre. Thrombosis of the IJV may be the only clue to the presence of adjacent malignancies like anaplastic carcinoma and follicular carcinoma of the thyroid. In patients with disseminated adenocarcinoma from an unknown primary, IJV thrombosis is associated with a poor prognosis.[53]

Masses in the posterior triangle

Given the paucity of structures in the posterior triangle, it is not surprising that the differential diagnosis of lesions at this site is limited. The lesions commonly encountered are:

Lymphatic malformation (cystic hygroma)

In infants these are commonly seen in the posterior triangle and in the cervicothoracic junction. The role of ultrasound and the ultrasound features have been discussed earlier in this chapter.

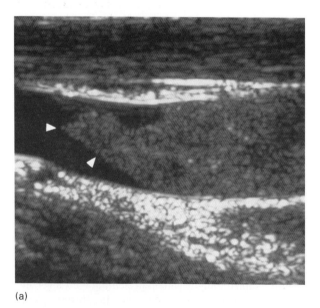
(a)

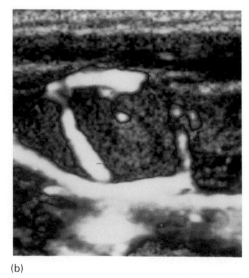
(b)

Figure 5.25 – Longitudinal sonogram of the internal jugular vein (a) showing an echogenic thrombus (arrowheads). Note the marked vascularity in (b), suggesting that this is a tumour thrombus.

Haemangioma

After the masseter muscle, the trapezius is the most common site for a head and neck intramuscular haemangioma. The ultrasound features have been described above.

Lipoma

The posterior triangle is a common site for large head and neck lipomas. Infiltrating lipomas rarely occur in the head and neck.[54] However, in patients with Madelung's disease (characterised by the presence of multiple, symmetrical, unencapsulated, large fatty accumulations diffusely involving the cervical and dorsal regions) the role of ultrasound is limited. MRI or non-contrast CT is necessary to evaluate precisely the extent of the fatty infiltration and the presence of any other incidental lesion in the neck.[55]

Liposarcoma

Liposarcomas, like lipomas, are relatively uncommon tumours in the head and neck. They do not arise from pre-existing lipomas, but from lipoblasts or totipotential mesenchyme within or adjacent to muscular and fascial structures.[15] The presence of ill-defined edges and heterogeneous internal architecture in a fatty tumour may suggest the diagnosis, but there are no obvious ultrasound features. CT or MRI is indicated to evaluate the extent, adjacent infiltration and internal architecture of these tumours. The attenuation of fat elements on CT is typically higher than that of subcutaneous fat, however these measurements are not reliable in tumours less than 2 cm in size.[56,57]

Nerve sheath tumours

Nerve sheath tumours arising from the cervical nerve roots present as masses in the posterior triangle and may be mistaken for lymph nodes which are more common at this site. The ultrasound features are discussed above.

Third branchial cleft cyst

A third branchial cleft cyst arises from the third branchial apparatus and presents as a painless fluctuant mass in the posterior triangle. It must be differentiated from the more common second BCC which is located in the posterior aspect of the submandibular region at the angle of the mandible and may encroach into the posterior triangle when it is large. If the lesion is centred in the posterior triangle then it is probably a third BCC.[3] The ultrasound features are similar to those of the second BCC discussed above.

Lymph nodes

Tuberculous and metastatic nodes (particularly from nasopharyngeal carcinoma) have a predilection for this site. Tuberculous nodes are frequently matted and show intranodal necrosis with adjacent oedema of the soft tissues or abscess formation.[58] These features help to distinguish them from metastatic nodes.

Miscellaneous neck masses

Thymic cyst

The congenital form of thymic cyst is rare. It arises from the thymopharyngeal duct. When acquired, these cysts are thought to develop as either inflammation or cystic degeneration of thymic remnants. They may be present anywhere from the angle of the mandible to the superior mediastinum adjacent to the carotid sheath. A connection with mediastinal thymic tissue may be present. They usually present as a painless mass. Two thirds of the cases occur in the first decade and the remaining third in the second and third decades.[3]

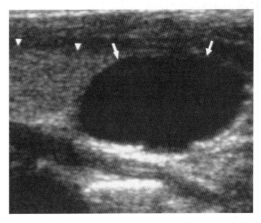

Figure 5.26 – Longitudinal sonogram showing a cystic lesion (arrows) below and separate from the thyroid gland (arrowheads). Note the anechoic nature. At this location the differential diagnosis includes a thymic cyst or a parathyroid cyst.

There are no specific ultrasound features of a thymic cyst, but it should be included in the differential diagnosis of a cyst below the level of the thyroid (Figure 5.26). A parathyroid cyst is the most common differential diagnosis, and its differentiation by ultrasound may also be difficult. Parathyroid cysts contain high parathormone and low T3, T4 levels. As thymic cysts are similar in location to the third and fourth BCC, they were previously considered to be a variant of BCC.

Bowel loops and mesentery

'Pull up surgery' in patients with hypopharyngeal, laryngeal and oesophageal cancer may confuse the inexperienced sonologist. Free jejunal autotransplantation is increasingly used as a surgical treatment for hypopharyngeal cancer. Ultrasound clearly identifies the peristaltic bowel (Figure 5.27) and the mesentery with its vascular arcades and lymph nodes.[59] It is important to recognise these structures to avoid mistaking them for pathology.

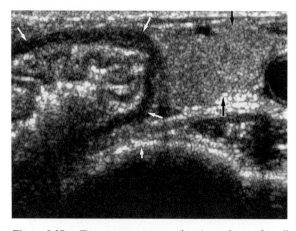

Figure 5.27 – Transverse sonogram showing a loop of small bowel (large white arrows) adjacent to the thyroid (black arrows), anterior to the vertebral body (small white arrow). The appearances are those of a jejunal pull-up.

Laryngocele

Laryngocele occurs when the laryngeal ventricle is functionally obstructed by increased intraglottic pressures arising from excessive coughing or playing a musical instrument. Obstruction due to postinflammatory stenosis, trauma or tumour is less common.[3] Patients commonly present with hoarseness of voice and neck swelling. Less commonly they may present with stridor, dysphagia, sore throat and pain.

ULTRASOUND FEATURES[60]

- Internal (simple) laryngoceles are echo-free, well-defined structures inside the thyroid cartilage.

- External (mixed) laryngoceles have an additional cystic mass outside the laryngeal skeleton (Figure 5.28) at the thyrohyoid membrane which is connected through the thyrohyoid membrane to the intralaryngeal component.

- When a laryngocele is infected the echoes within it are mixed and the walls may appear thickened.

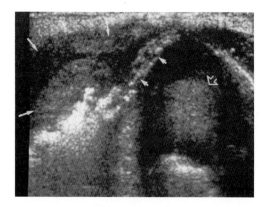

Figure 5.28 – Transverse sonogram of an external (mixed) laryngocele showing a collection (large arrows) and debris (open arrow) on either side of the laryngeal skeleton (small arrows).

References

1. Ying M, Ahuja A, Brook F, Brown B, Metreweli C. Sonographic appearances and distribution of normal cervical lymph nodes in Chinese population. *J Ultrasound Med* 1996; **15:** 431–436.

2. Ahuja AT, Leung SF, Teo PM *et al.* Submental metastases from nasopharyngeal carcinoma. *Clin Radiol* 1999; **54:** 25–28.

3. Harnsberger RH. *Handbook of Head and Neck Imaging,* 2nd edn. St Louis: Mosby-Year Book, 1995; pp 199–223.

4. New GB, Erich JB. Dermoid cyst of the head and neck. *Surg Gynecol Obstet* 1937; **65:** 48.

5. Reynolds JH, Wolinski AP. Sonographic appearance of branchial cysts. *Clin Radiol* 1993; **2:** 109–110.

6. Ahuja AT, Yang WT, Metreweli C. Ultrasound of the salivary glands. *Indian J Radiol Imaging* 1998; **8(1):** 57–64.

7. Ahuja AT, Yang WT, King W, Metreweli C. Ultrasound and guided fine needle aspiration cytology in the submandibular triangle. *S Afr J Radiol* 1997; **2(3):** 8–13.

8. Gritzmann N. Sonography of the salivary glands. *AJR* 1989; **53:** 161–166.

9. Harnsberger RH. *Handbook of Head and Neck Imaging,* 2nd edn. St Louis: Mosby-Year Book, 1995; pp 120–149.

10. Ahuja A, Ying M, King W, Metreweli C. A practical approach to ultrasound of cervical lymph nodes. *J Laryngol Otol* 1997; **111:** 245–256.

11. Ahuja A, Ying M, Yang WT, Evans R, King W, Metreweli C. The use of sonography in differentiating cervical lymphomatous nodes from cervical metastatic lymph nodes. *Clin Radiol* 1996; **51:** 186–190.

12. Ahuja AT, Loke TKL, Mok CO, Chow LTC, Metreweli C. Ultrasound of Kimura's disease. *Clin Radiol* 1995; **50:** 170–173.

13. Benhoff DF, Wood JW. Infiltrating lipomata of the head and neck. *Laryngoscope* 1978; **88:** 839.

14. Ahuja AT, King AD, Kew J, King W, Metreweli C. Head and neck lipomas: ultrasound appearances. *Am J Neuroradiol* 1998; **19:** 505–508.

15. Reede DL. Nodal and non-nodal neck masses. Part II. Non-nodal neck masses. In: Som PM, Curtin HD, Holliday RA, eds. *Special Course in Head and Neck Radiology.* Radiological Society of North America 1996; 75–86.

16. Weismann JL. Nonnodal masses of the neck. In: Som PM, Curtin HD, eds. *Head and Neck Imaging,* 3rd edn. St Louis: Mosby-Year Book, 1996; pp 794–822.

17. Bruneton JN, Fenart D. Other cervical sites. In: Bruneton JN, ed. *Ultrasonography of the Neck.* Berlin: Springer-Verlag, 1987; pp 93–106.

18. Baatenburg de Jong RJ, Rongen RJ, Lameris JS, Knegt P, Verwoerd CDA. Ultrasound characteristics of thyroglossal duct anomalies. *ORL* 1993; **55:** 299–302.

19. Ahuja AT, Ng CF, King W, Metreweli C. Solitary cystic nodal metastasis from occult papillary carcinoma of the thyroid mimicking a branchial cyst: a potential pitfall. *Clin Radiol* 1998; **53:** 61–63.

20. Siegel MJ, Glazer HS, St Amour TE *et al.* Lymphangiomas in children: MR imaging. *Radiology* 1989; **170:** 467–470.

21. Zadvinskis DP, Benson MT, Kerr HH *et al.* Congenital malformations of the cervicothoracic lymphatic system: embryology and pathogenesis. *Radiographics* 1992; **12:** 1175–1189.

22. Singh S, Baboo ML, Pathak LC. Cystic lymphangioma in children: report of 32 cases including lesions at rare sites. *Surgery* 1971; **69:** 947.

23. Kalifa G, Poncin J, Sellier N. Cervical pathologies in children. In: Bruneton JN, ed. *Ultrasonography of the Neck.* Berlin: Springer-Verlag, 1987; pp 107–113.

24. Noujaim S, Arpasi P, Bennett DF, Bohdiewicz P, Dworkin H. Imaging thyroglossal duct anomalies. *The Radiologist* 1997; **4(5):** 235–241.

25. Wadsworth DT, Siegel MJ. Thyroglossal duct cysts: variability of sonographic findings. *AJR* 1994; **163:** 1475–1477.

26. Friedman AP, Haller JO, Goodman JD, Nagar H. Sonographic evaluation of non-inflammatory neck masses in children. *Radiology* 1983; **147:** 693–697.

27. Kraus R, Han BK, Babcock DS, Oestreich AE. Sonography of neck masses in children. *AJR* 1986; **146:** 609–613.

28. Ahuja AT, King AD, Metreweli C. Thyroglossal duct cysts: sonographic appearances in adults. *AJNR,* 1999; **20:** 579–582.

29. Hayes LL, Marlow SF Jr. Papillary carcinoma arising in a thyroglossal duct cyst. *Laryngoscope* 1968; **78:** 2189–2193.

30. Boswell WC. Thyroglossal duct carcinoma. *Am Surgeon* 1994; **60:** 650–655.

31. Pelausa EO, Forte V. Sistrunk revisited: a ten year review of revision thyroglossal duct surgery at Toronto's Hospital for Sick Children. *J Otolaryngol* 1989; **18:** 325–333.

32. Yang WT, Ahuja AT, Metreweli C. Role of ultrasound in the imaging of parotid swellings. *S Afr J Radiol* March 1996, 18–22.

33. Bradley MJ, Ahuja A, Metreweli C. Sonographic evaluation of the parotid ducts: its use in tumour localization. *Br J Radiol* 1991; **64:** 1092–1095.

34. Smyth AG. Botulinum toxin treatment of bilateral masseteric hypertrophy. *Br J Oral Maxillofac Surg* 1994; **32:** 29–33.

35. Harnsberger RH. *Handbook of Head and Neck Imaging,* 2nd edn. St Louis: Mosby-Year Book, 1995; pp 60–74.

36. Emery PJ, Salama NY. Congenital preauricular sinus. A study of 131 cases seen over a ten year period. *Int J Paediatr Otorhinolaryngol* 1981; **3:** 205–218.

37. Rossiter JL, Hendrix RA, Tom LWC *et al.* Intramuscular haemangioma of the head and neck. *Otolaryngol Head Neck Surg* 1993; **108:** 18.

38. Batsakis JG. Tumours of the head and neck: clinical and pathological considerations. Baltimore: Williams and Wilkins, 1979; p 294.

39. Shallow TA, Eger SA, Wagner FB. Primary haemangiomatous tumours of skeletal muscle. *Ann Surg* 1944; **119:** 700.

40. Yonetsu K, Nakayama E, Hunihir M *et al.* Magnetic resonance imaging of oral and maxillofacial angiomas. *Oral Surg Oral Med Oral Path* 1993; **16:** 783–789.

41. Derchi LE, Balconi G, De Flaviis L, Olivia A, Rosso F. Sonographic appearance of haemangiomas of skeletal muscle. *J Ultrasound Med* 1989; **8:** 263–267.

42. Yang WT, Ahuja A, Metreweli C. Sonographic features of head and neck hemangiomas and vascular malformations: review of 23 patients. *J Ultrasound Med* 1997; **16:** 39–44.

43. Pratt LW. Familial carotid body tumours. *Arch Otolaryngol* 1973; **97:** 334.

44. Rush BF, Jr. Familial carotid body tumours. *Ann Surg* 1963; **157:** 633.

45. Lack EE. Paragangliomas of the head and neck region: a clinical study of 69 patients. *Cancer* 1977; **39:** 397.

46. Stull MA, Moser RP Jr, Kransdorf MJ *et al.* Magnetic resonance appearance of peripheral nerve sheath tumours. *Skel Radiol* 1991; **20:** 9–14.

47. Barnes L, Peel RL, Verbin RS. Tumors of the nervous system. In: Barnes L, ed. *Surgical Pathology of the Head and Neck*. New York: Marcel Dekker, 1985; pp 659–724.

48. Fornage BD. Soft tissue masses. In: Fornage BD, ed. *Musculoskeletal Ultrasound*. New York: Churchill Livingstone, 1995; pp 21–42.

49. King AD, Ahuja AT, King W, Metreweli C. Sonography of peripheral nerve tumors of the neck. *AJR* 1997; **169:** 1695–1698.

50. Hoddick WK, Callen PW, Filly RA, Mahony BS, Edwards MB. Ultrasound evaluation of benign sciatic nerve sheath tumours. *J Ultrasound Med* 1984; **3:** 505–507.

51. Chinn DH, Filly RA, Callen PW. Unusual ultrasonographic appearance of a solid schwannoma. *J Clin Ultrasound* 1982; **10:** 243–245.

52. Fornage BD. Sonography of the peripheral nerves of the extremities. *Radiol Med* 1993; **5:** 162–167.

53. Lam WM, Ahuja AT, Mok CO, Metreweli C. Spontaneous internal jugular vein thrombosis associated with adenocarcinoma of unknown primary. *Hong Kong Med J* 1995; **1:** 258–260.

54. Batsakis JG. *Tumours of the Head and Neck: Clinical and Pathological Considerations*. Baltimore: Williams and Wilkins, 1979; pp 240–250.

55. Ahuja AT, King AD, Chan ESY *et al*. Madelung's disease: distribution of cervical fat and pre-operative evaluation as seen with ultrasound, MR and CT. *AJNR* 1998; **19:** 707–710.

56. Friedman AC. Computed tomography of abdominal fatty masses. *Radiology* 1981; **139:** 415.

57. Hansen GE. Computed tomography diagnosis of renal angiomyolipoma. *Radiology* 1978; **128:** 789.

58. Ahuja A, Ying M, Evans R, King W, Metreweli C. The application of ultrasound criteria for malignancy in differentiating tuberculous cervical adenitis from metastatic nasopharyngeal carcinoma. *Clin Radiol* 1995; **50:** 391–395.

59. Ahuja A, Zekri A, Davey IC, Mok CO, King W, Metreweli C. Ultrasound characteristics of jejunal flap used in pharyngoesophageal reconstruction. *J Clin Ultrasound* 1995; **23(1):** 38–41.

60. Baatenburg de Jong RJ, Rongen RJ, Lameris JS, Knegt P, Verwoerd CDA. Ultrasound in the diagnosis of laryngoceles. *ORL* 1993; **55:** 290–293.

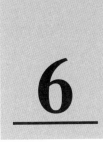

6

THE LARYNX

Dr Eric Loveday

Anatomy and sonographic anatomy
Examination technique
Vocal folds
Clinical applications

Introduction

The larynx is an important organ occupying a central position in the neck. It is an air-containing structure whose elements may become heavily calcified, and as such might be regarded as a less than ideal candidate for ultrasound examination. Despite its anatomical complexity, however, many of its component parts lie superficially in the neck and have good inherent soft tissue contrast, and are therefore ideally suited to examination by high resolution ultrasound. Non-invasive assessment of vocal cord movement is possible, and in comparison with other cross-sectional imaging modalities there are obvious advantages in terms of cost and patient tolerance.

This chapter will illustrate the anatomy and sonographic anatomy of the larynx. The strengths and weakness of the sonographic approach will be discussed, along with potential clinical applications.

Anatomy and sonographic anatomy

The larynx is undoubtedly a complex organ, and a detailed discussion of its anatomy and function is beyond the scope of this text; hence, only those aspects of anatomy that lend themselves to sonographic evaluation will be portrayed.

The larynx plays a vital part in speech, protection of the aerodigestive tract and swallowing. Both intrinsic activity and movement of the larynx as a whole occur to varying degrees in all of these activities.

The basic elements are the three parts of the skeleton bound together by ligaments and muscles. Supported within this framework are the cardinal functional components – the vocal folds and the epiglottis. The skeleton comprises the hyoid bone and the thyroid and cricoid cartilages (Figure 6.1). The hyoid bone calcifies early in life and is invariably sonopaque, thus providing a useful anatomic landmark. The thyroid and cricoid cartilages are predominantly composed of hyaline cartilage. This has a propensity to calcify to a variable degree, unlike the elastic cartilage of the epiglottis, which is invariably sonolucent. The arytenoid cartilages, which are also composed of hyaline cartilage, sit on the posterior lamina of the cricoid cartilage.

The laryngeal skeleton is supported by the thyrohyoid and cricothyroid ligaments (Figure 6.2); the latter is overlain by the thin cricothyroid muscle. The thyroepiglottic and hyoepiglottic ligaments tether the base and body respectively of the epiglottis, whose superior rim, together with the aryepiglottic folds, forms the upper limit of the supraglottic larynx.

The oblique line on the outer surface of the laryngeal cartilage forms the attachment for the cricopharyngeus muscle extending posteriorly and, for the first layer of strap muscles, the sternothyroid extending inferiorly

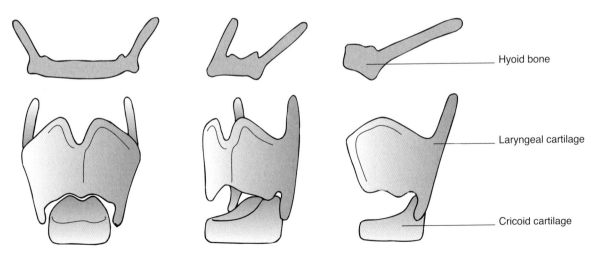

Figure 6.1 – The skeleton of the larynx in frontal, oblique and lateral views.

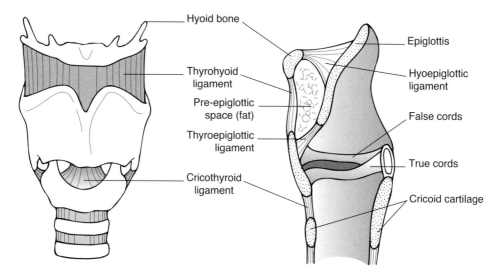

Figure 6.2 – Anterior view and midline sagittal section of the larynx, showing the principal ligaments, true and false cords and pre-epiglottic space.

and the thyrohyoid superiorly (Figure 6.3). The second layer of strap muscles constitutes the omohyoid posteriorly and the sternohyoid anteriorly; unlike the deep layer these do not attach directly to the laryngeal cartilage (Figures 6.4, 6.5).

Within the larynx are the true and false vocal folds (Figures 6.2, 6.6). The true folds are composed mainly of intrinsic skeletal muscle and are predominantly echo-poor (Figures 6.7, 6.8).

The remainder of the interior of the larynx is largely composed of fatty connective tissue containing vessels, lymphatics, nerves and some smaller intrinsic muscles. This fat has a characteristic finely echogenic appearance on ultrasound. Anatomically, this is the paraglottic space (Figure 6.8), and it is important to realise that this space is continuous anteriorly and superiorly with the pre-epiglottic space (Figure 6.2), a fact which may readily be appreciated on ultrasound (Figure 6.9).

Examination technique

When examining the larynx it is essential, as with any organ, to follow a systematic method. The order in which the various elements are examined is of less importance than the principle of undertaking a thorough evaluation.

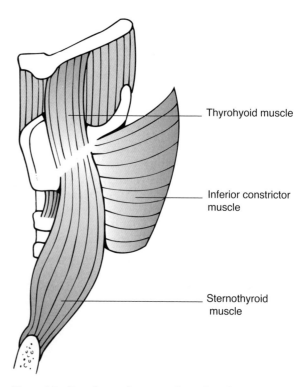

Figure 6.3 – Deep layer of strap muscles, in lateral view, attaching to the oblique line on the surface of the thyroid cartilage.

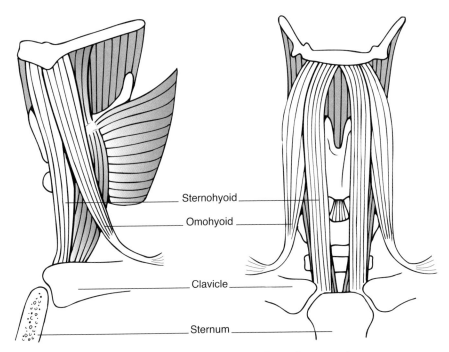

Figure 6.4 – Lateral and frontal views of the larynx, showing the superficial layer of strap muscles.

The larynx itself may present a variable appearance, and its size may differ markedly between individuals. Hence anatomical landmarks assume an important role. The most constant sonographic landmark is the hyoid bone, which is easily identified in the midline in longitudinal section and casts a dense acoustic shadow (see for example Figure 6.9b). The surgically important pre-epiglottic space is well seen in this section, and should be examined also in transverse section. Moving off the midline in parasagittal section, the strap muscles are seen as they attach to the inferior border of the hyoid, and can be traced inferiorly. They have a characteristic appearance in this section, forming a broad, finely striated, sonolucent longitudinal stripe beneath which the laryngeal cartilage can be identified (Figures 6.5, 6.7, 6.9c). The cricoid cartilage should be identified, as should the mucosa/air interface beneath it (Figure 6.7), as far as calcification permits.

Vocal folds

Although the parasagittal section displays certain elements of laryngeal anatomy well, the vocal folds produce a very variable echopattern which is difficult to reproduce. Movement can occasionally be assessed in this projection, but is again poorly reproducible as the amount of movement seen will depend on which part of the cord (anterior or posterior) intersects the sound beam. It is important to note that the true vocal folds overlie echo-poor muscle, while the false cords overlie echogenic fat and, on occasion, variable bright echoes due to the unpredictable appearance of the laryngeal vestibule.

This fact is of use when identifying the vocal folds in transverse section; again the vocal folds have a distinctive appearance being echo-poor, while at the level of the false cords, echogenic paraglottic fat is seen (Figures 6.8, 6.11).

The midline transverse sonogram as depicted in Figure 6.10 is of most value in assessing *movement* of the vocal folds, as it allows the movement of the two sides to be compared. Although the free edge of the fold has a poor reflective angle to the sound wave in this projection, detail is adequate to assess movement. Even in the most heavily calcified larynx this view is usually possible, and often the arytenoid cartilages can be seen, further enhancing assessment of symmetry.

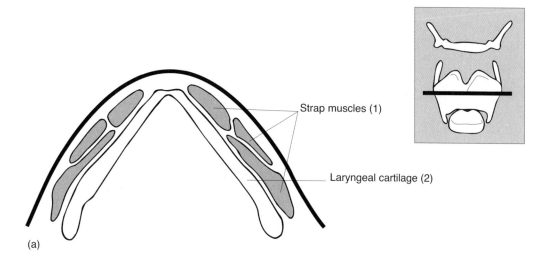

Strap muscles (1)

Laryngeal cartilage (2)

(a)

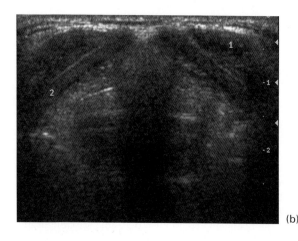

(b)

Figure 6.5 – (a) Cross-section through the laryngeal cartilage showing the appearance of the strap muscles. *(Note: The boxed diagram in this and subsequent illustrations represents the laryngeal skeleton, the heavy line indicating the plane of section or the position of the footprint of the ultrasound probe.)* (b) Corresponding sonogram. Note that the sonographic appearance varies according to the level of section, and between individuals.

Vocal fold movement is best observed during quiet breathing, during which the normal vocal folds will abduct on inspiration and relax towards the midline on expiration. Attempts to assess voluntary movements such as phonation are hampered by the gross movements of the larynx that these manoeuvres provoke.

The transverse off-centre view may be used to provide better depiction of the surface of the vocal fold, but is more often affected by cartilage calcification.

Clinical applications

Laryngeal cancer

The fundamental principle of pre-operative staging of laryngeal cancer is thorough clinical and endoscopic examination, supplemented by imaging where appropriate, usually CT or MRI. A plain chest radiograph is usually performed, particularly with a view to ruling out a synchronous bronchial neoplasm.

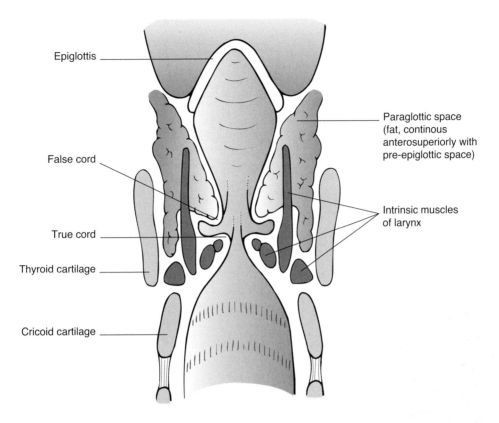

Epiglottis

Paraglottic space
(fat, continous
anterosuperiorly with
pre-epiglottic space)

False cord

Intrinsic muscles
of larynx

True cord

Thyroid cartilage

Cricoid cartilage

Figure 6.6 – Coronal section through the larynx showing the predominantly muscular composition of the true vocal cords, and the fatty connective tissue of the paraglottis and false cords.

Smaller tumours are adequately assessed by flexible fibreoptic nasolaryngoscopy, examination under anaesthesia and biopsy, without any need for further imaging. With increasing tumour size, however, the likelihood of deep invasion increases, and imaging has a role in the detection of deep spread to the paraglottic space, pre-epiglottic space and laryngeal cartilages. Ultrasound is capable of extremely high resolution of superficial structures, and is largely unaffected by patient movement; hence its potential role merits closer inspection.

Those parts of the larynx which best lend themselves to ultrasonographic assessment are those structures which lie superficially and anteriorly, particularly the laryngeal cartilages, ligaments, pre-epiglottic space and paraglottis. Conversely, posterior structures which are largely obscured by the air column are less well suited.

These include the upper epiglottis and aryepiglottic folds, although these are generally well assessed clinically.

The *pre-epiglottic space* is an important surgical blind spot as it is impossible to assess either clinically or endoscopically. As indicated above, it is anatomically continuous with the paraglottis, with its rich network of lymphatics, and hence is an important route of spread of supraglottic tumours in particular. Tumour spreading in this manner is well detected, being echo-poor in contrast with the finely echogenic fat of the pre-epiglottic space and paraglottis (Figure 6.11).

The detection of *extralaryngeal spread* is of great importance in pre-treatment staging. Glottic tumours have a propensity to invade through the cricothyroid membrane while both glottic and supraglottic tumours may

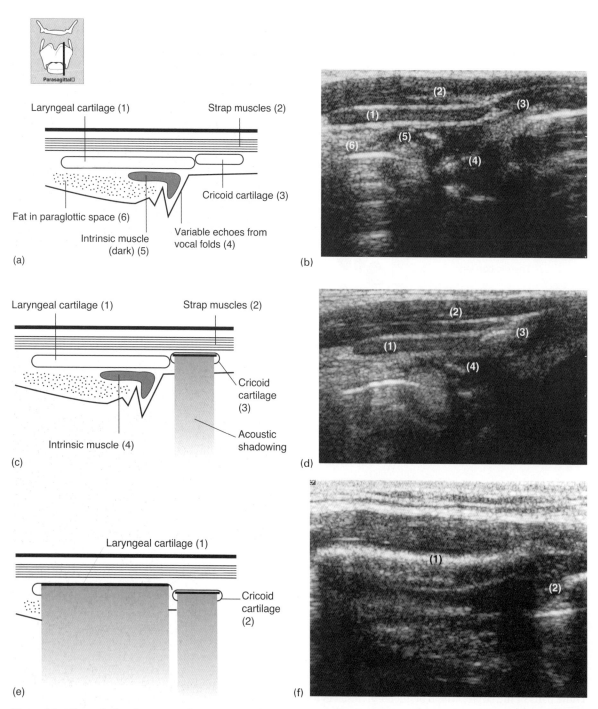

Parasagittal

Laryngeal cartilage (1)   Strap muscles (2)

Fat in paraglottic space (6)

Intrinsic muscle (dark) (5)   Cricoid cartilage (3)

Variable echoes from vocal folds (4)

(a)

(b)

Laryngeal cartilage (1)   Strap muscles (2)

Cricoid cartilage (3)

Acoustic shadowing

Intrinsic muscle (4)

(c)

(d)

Laryngeal cartilage (1)

Cricoid cartilage (2)

(e)

(f)

Figure 6.7 – Parasagittal and corresponding sonograms showing the variable appearance of the laryngeal cartilage. (a) & (b) Fully sonolucent cartilage. The overlying strap muscles form a sonolucent stripe with fine longitudinal striations. The internal structures of the larynx are clearly visible. Note that the free edge of the vocal fold has a variable appearance in longitudinal section. (c) & (d) Often the cartilage is partially calcified causing variable loss of visualisation of intralaryngeal structures. (e) and (f) On occasion the majority of the cartilage is calcified, limiting the view of intralaryngeal structures.

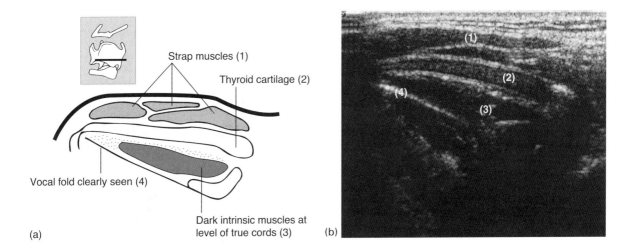

(a)
Strap muscles (1)
Thyroid cartilage (2)
Vocal fold clearly seen (4)
Dark intrinsic muscles at
level of true cords (3)

(b)

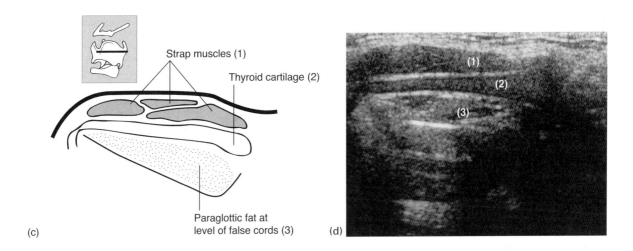

(c)
Strap muscles (1)
Thyroid cartilage (2)
Paraglottic fat at
level of false cords (3)

(d)

Figure 6.8 – (a) Transverse off-centre section at the level of the vocal folds and (b) corresponding sonogram. Note the echo-poor nature of the intrinsic muscles at this level. Compare the corresponding sections (c) and (d) at a slightly higher level, where the paraglottic fat is more echogenic.

directly invade the thyroid cartilage. The high spatial resolution of good quality ultrasound units lends itself to the early detection of this mode of spread (Figure 6.12).

Involvement of the *vocal folds* by laryngeal tumours is another important aspect of staging, impaired mobility or fixity denoting T3 stage depending on whether the tumour is supraglottic or glottic respectively. The vast majority of cases are well assessed endoscopically, but ultrasound may make a contribution on occasions where a large supraglottic tumour obscures the view of the cords, or the patient cannot tolerate the endoscopic examination.

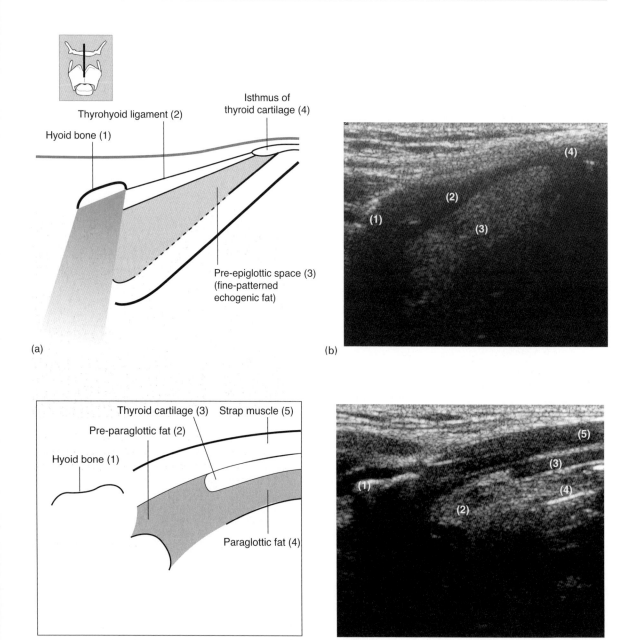

Figure 6.9 – (a) Midline sagittal section through the upper larynx showing the pre–epiglottic space (c.f. Figure 6.3). (b) Corresponding sonogram. If the probe is moved laterally (c), the upper part of the laryngeal cartilage comes into view, and the continuity of the pre-epiglottic and paraglottic fat may be appreciated (c.f. Figure 6.7 a & b).

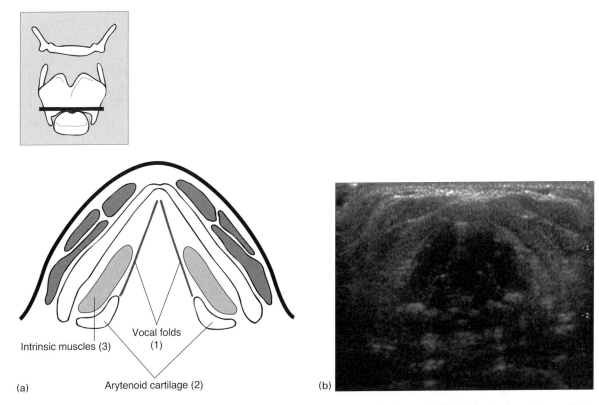

Figure 6.10 – Midline transverse section (a) and corresponding sonogram (b) through the vocal folds. In the sonolucent larynx, this is the best view for assessing movement as symmetry can be observed. The arytenoid cartilages may be seen but their appearance is poorly reproducible (see Figure 6.5 (b) for corresponding sonogram). The free edges of the vocal folds form a poor reflecting angle with the sound beam in this projection, but are more readily perceived during the real-time examination.

The frequency of cervical *lymph node spread* increases with increasing T-stage, with supraglottic tumours having a particular tendency to early spread. Increasingly head and neck sonologists are becoming involved in nodal staging of head and neck cancers. The value of imaging depends to some degree upon whether local practice dictates a surgical or radiotherapeutic approach to the node-positive neck.

The role of ultrasound in laryngeal carcinoma remains to be defined. It is unlikely to gain acceptance as a sole imaging modality, but there is certainly evidence for a complementary role with clinical examination and CT or MRI. Any sonologist regularly engaging in cervical lymph node staging should familiarise himself with the sonographic anatomy of the larynx. In so doing he should be able to contribute to the staging of known primary laryngeal tumours, and usefully assess any

laryngeal invasion by tumours arising in neighbouring structures.

Vocal fold mobility in children

Few young children will tolerate either direct or indirect laryngoscopy, and the assessment of vocal fold mobility in the child presenting with hoarseness or stridor poses a significant challenge to the ENT surgeon. Ultrasound, using the methods described above, is well suited to non-invasive assessment of vocal fold function and symmetry – the more so since the juvenile larynx is predominantly sonolucent, containing as it does little or no calcification. There is, however, little in the way of published evidence at the present time to indicate adequate sensitivity or specificity for this technique.

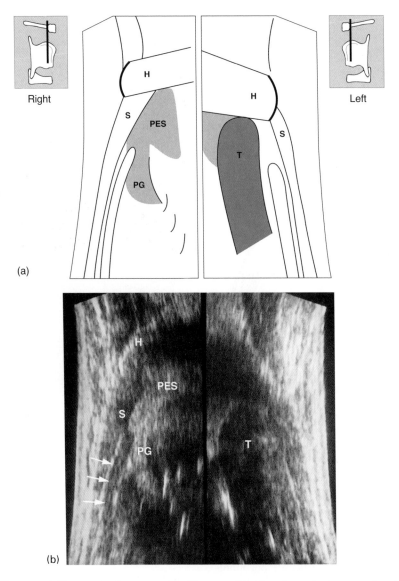

Figure 6.11 – (a) Diagram and (b) corresponding sonograms. The pre-epiglottic and paraglottic spaces. Longitudinal, coronal sonograms of the right (normal) and left (abnormal) sides, mounted opposite each other in each case to simulate a coronal image of the whole larynx. On the left side, tumour (T) arising within the larynx invades the paraglottic space (PG) and extends superiorly into the pre-epiglottic space (PES). (H = hyoid bone with acoustic shadow. S = strap muscles. Arrows = outer surface of thyroid cartilage.) Reproduced with permission of the Editor, *Clinical Radiology*.

Conclusion

In this chapter the anatomy, sonographic anatomy and method of sonographic examination of the larynx have been illustrated, and the potential clinical applications, strengths and weaknesses have been discussed. The capacity of ultrasound to demonstrate subtle abnormalities in this region is due to its high spatial resolution and dynamic nature.

In examining the larynx, ultrasound should properly be regarded as a complementary imaging modality whose benefits include high patient acceptability and low cost. It is suggested that every head and neck radiolo-

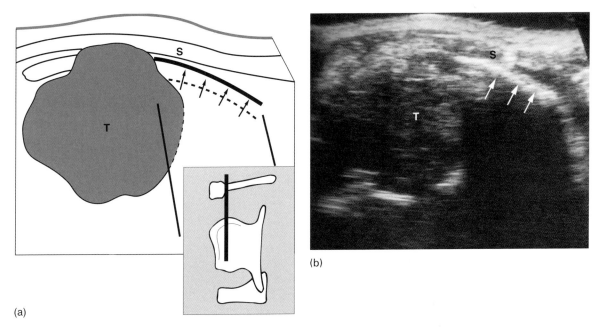

(a)

(b)

Figure 6.12 – (a) Diagram and (b) corresponding sonogram. Longitudinal section through thyroid cartilage. A large supraglottic tumour (T) is shown invading through the thyroid cartilage. The outer surface of the cartilage forms a reflecting line (arrows) which is interrupted by the extralaryngeal tumour spread. Note that the calcified inferior part of the thyroid cartilage in this case casts an acoustic shadow, the edges of which are indicated by the straight lines on the diagram. Reproduced with permission of the Editor, *Clinical Radiology*.

gist should familiarise himself with the sonographic anatomy of the larynx, and explore the value of this technique.

References

1. Bears OH, Henson DE, Hutter RVP, Myers MH, eds. *American Joint Committee on Cancer: Manual for staging of cancer*, 3rd edn. Philadelphia: JB Lippincott, 1988; pp 39–41.

2. Erkan M, Tolu I, Aslan T, Güney E. Ultrasonography in laryngeal cancers. *J Laryngol Otol* 1993; **107:** 65–68.

3. Friedmann EM. Role of ultrasound in the assessment of vocal fold function in infants and children. *Ann Otol Rhinol Laryngol* 1997; **106:** 199–209.

4. Gritzmann N, Traxler M, Grasl M, Pavelka R. Advanced laryngeal cancer: Sonographic assessment. *Radiology* 1989; **171:** 171–175.

5. Johnson JT, Myers EN. Cervical lymph node disease in laryngeal cancer. In: Silver CE, ed. *Laryngeal Cancer*. New York: Thieme, 1991; pp 22–26.

6. Loevner LA, Yousem DM, Montone KT, Weber R, Chalian AA, Weinstein GS. Can radiologists accurately predict preepiglottic space invasion with MR imaging? *AJR* 1997; **169:** 1681–1687.

7. Loveday EJ, Bleach NR, Van Hasselt CA, Metreweli C. Ultrasound imaging in laryngeal cancer: a preliminary study. *Clin Radiol* 1994; **49:** 676–682.

8. Phelps PD. Carcinoma of the larynx – the role of imaging in staging and pre-treatment assessments. *Clin Radiol* 1992; **46:** 77–83.

9. Rothberg S, Noyek AM, Freeman JL, Steinhardt MI, Stoll S, Goldfinger M. Thyroid cartilage imaging with diagnostic ultrasound. *Arch Otolaryngol Head and Neck Surg* 1986; **112:** 503–515.

10. Sanghvi V. The new combined surgical approach for cancer involving the base-of-tongue-supraglottic complex. *Laryngoscope* 1994; **104:** 725–730.

11. Zbaren P, Becker M, Lang H. Pretherapeutic staging of hypopharyngeal carcinoma. Clinical findings, computed tomography, and magnetic resonance imaging compared with histopathologic evaluation. *Arch Otolaryngol Head & Neck Surg* 1997; **123:** 908–913.

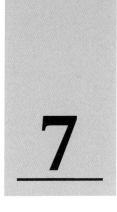

7

WHAT THE SURGEON
NEEDS TO KNOW, AND WHY

DW Patton, KC Silvester

The clinical characteristics of a lump
Establishing a tissue diagnosis
Malignant lumps in the neck
Does improved imaging result in a
    better outcome for the patient?

Introduction

A surgeon working in the head and neck area is frequently asked to see lumps or swellings presenting in that region. In the past, the diagnosis depended on an accurate history followed by a thorough clinical examination. On the basis of these, the surgeon would then select those investigations which would confirm or refute the clinical diagnosis. The surgical management of the case was thus determined. An investigation would only be justified if the findings would influence the decision on the type of treatment to be prescribed.

Although sophisticated imaging techniques now exist, the history and clinical examination still remain the most important means of diagnosing neck and facial 'lumps'. In this chapter, we outline what the surgeon would ideally like to know about a lump before any treatment is undertaken. We focus mainly on lumps in the neck as this is the area where there is the greatest controversy. In particular, we will stress the importance of accurate assessment of the regional lymph nodes in head and neck cancer, as this largely determines the surgical management of the case and the outcome for the patient.

The clinical characteristics of a lump

In the past, when imaging procedures were unsophisticated, surgeons would pride themselves on their ability to elicit subtle clinical signs. The ability to do this depended on a long clinical apprenticeship and skilled clinical teachers. Invariably, the ability of surgeons to come to the correct diagnosis, based on a clinical examination alone, varied considerably. Many would argue that shorter training and a greater reliance on sophisticated imaging techniques have eroded surgeons' abilities to elicit the less obvious clinical signs. Nevertheless, surgeons still rely on their ability to detect the clinical characteristics of a lump and reach a diagnosis.

Having taken the history, there are a number of physical signs which a surgeon tries to elicit by feeling a neck lump. The characteristics of the lump in conjunction with its history may suggest the diagnosis. For example, a lump of 'rubbery' consistency might suggest Hodgkin's disease; a rock-hard lump which is fixed to the skin or deeper structures is likely to result

from malignant disease. Some lumps, particularly cystic hygroma, transilluminate brilliantly when a pen torch is pushed into the lump. If the lump is tender or hot, this suggests inflammation such as an abscess.

CLINICAL EXAMINATION OF A LUMP
Size
Site
Shape
Surface (smooth, craggy, etc.)
Edge (well-defined, diffuse, etc.)
Consistency (hard, rubbery, fluctuant, soft)
Is it tender?
Is it hot?
Is it fixed to skin?
Is it fixed to deep structures?
Is it pulsatile?
Does it transilluminate?
Are the regional lymph nodes enlarged?

After the surgeon has completed the examination he would hope to have some indication whether the mass is a swelling or lump, whether a lump is cystic or solid, and, if solid, whether it is inflammatory (such as a reactionary lymph node) or a tumour (Figure 7.1). If the lump is a tumour, then he would hope to have an indication whether it is benign or malignant.

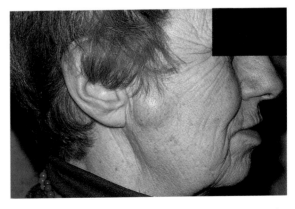

Figure 7.1 – A common diagnostic problem; the pre-auricular lump. Pre-operative imaging is generally very helpful in establishing a diagnosis. In this case the lump is a pleomorphic adenoma of the parotid salivary gland.

Establishing a tissue diagnosis

In the past, before the advent of imaging techniques such as CT and MRI, the only way a surgeon could obtain further information about the lump was by carrying out a biopsy. This was often an open biopsy which carried the risk, in malignant disease, of seeding the surrounding tissues. Radiographs might have been of some help if there was bone involvement. It was frequently necessary to carry out an operation to remove a lump with only a vague suspicion of what the final diagnosis might be. The areas which caused particular difficulty were lumps in the parotid salivary gland and lumps in the neck. The teaching had been that parotid lumps should not be biopsied because of the high risk of seeding or of damaging branches of the facial nerve. Only when the histopathology report became available was it apparent that the lump, thought to be benign, was in fact malignant. The operation carried out may have been inappropriate, and there may well have been residual disease. The outcome following a further, more radical resection would then not be as good as if a more radical procedure had been carried out in the first place. If, on the other hand, the lump had been thought to be malignant, and a radical resection had been performed, there would have been unnecessary morbidity had the lump been shown to be benign. This problem related mainly to the neck, where radical neck dissection was carried out for perceived spread of malignant disease from a primary tumour in the mouth or pharynx.

The advent of fine-needle aspiration techniques made it easier for a surgeon to obtain an indication of the nature of the lump pre-operatively. It depended, however, on the needle actually being in the lump when the sample was taken, and the availability of a pathologist experienced in the interpretation of the specimen. The interpretation of salivary tumours in particular was (and still is) challenging. There was also a debate whether fine-needle aspiration cytology (FNAC) could cause seeding of a malignant tumour or of benign tumours such as a pleomorphic adenoma of the salivary gland. However, the evidence was that the risk of seeding was very small or absent.

Malignant lumps in the neck

Nowhere in the head and neck is the accurate diagnosis of neck lumps more important than in the assessment of the neck nodes in head and neck cancer. 80% of cancers in the head and neck region are squamous cell carcinomas of the upper aerodigestive tract. The tumours spread by the lymphatics rather than blood, and the initial spread is therefore to the lymph nodes in the neck (Figure 7.2). The incidence and site of lymph node metastases in the neck vary with the site and size of the primary tumour. Generally, the overall incidence of neck node metastases in oral cancer is about 50%,[1] but it may be as high as 80% in nasopharyngeal carcinoma.

There is general agreement that the status of the neck nodes is the most important prognostic factor in head and neck cancer.[2] Moreover, the assessment of the neck nodes is critical in planning treatment, both surgery and radiotherapy. When nodal metastases exist at presentation or develop subsequently, cure rates decrease by around 50%. Extranodal spread, and the number of positive nodes, are the two histological factors that are of most importance for recurrence in the neck. The number of histologically positive nodes

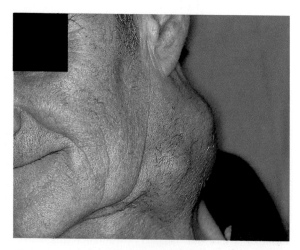

Figure 7.2 – A large malignant lymph node in the neck. The primary tumour was a squamous cell carcinoma of the tongue.

(more than three), extranodal spread of tumour, and lymph node metastases at multiple levels in the neck have also been shown to be important indicators for the risk of recurrence in the neck.[2]

HEAD AND NECK CANCER

1   The status of the neck nodes is the most important single prognostic factor in head and neck cancer.
2   The accurate staging of the neck nodes in cancer of the upper aerodigestive tract is an important factor in the planning of treatment.

Staging of the neck nodes in malignant disease

Not only is the accurate staging of the nodes essential for treatment planning, it is also the basis on which meaningful prospective studies can be carried out to enable the development of protocols and guidelines. This is essential to ensure that, for a particular tumour, at a particular site, and at a particular stage, the most effective treatment is given on the basis of the best available evidence (Figure 7.3). The staging is based on the TNM system; this depends on an assessment of the size of the primary tumour (T), the status of the regional lymph nodes (N) and the presence, or absence, of metastases (M). The staging of the lymph nodes is based on the size and number of nodes, and whether they are unilateral or bilateral.

UICC T STAGING OF THE PRIMARY TUMOUR IN ORAL CANCER (TNM SYSTEM)

TIS   Pre-invasive carcinoma (carcinoma in situ)
T0   No evidence of primary tumour
T1   Tumour 2 cm or less in its greatest dimension
T2   Tumour greater than 2 cm but less than 4 cm in its greatest dimension
T3   Tumour more than 4 cm but less than 6 cm in its greatest dimension
T4   Tumour greater than 6 cm in dimension, or a tumour with direct extension to bone or muscle

---

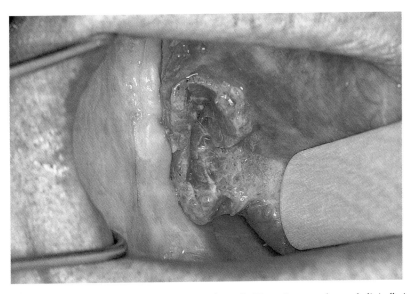

Figure 7.3 – A T2 squamous cell carcinoma of the tongue/floor of mouth. No nodes were detected clinically in the neck. The management of the neck in this situation remains controversial. Current advances in imaging techniques may influence the surgical management.

UICC TNM STAGING FOR NECK NODE METASTASES IN ORAL CANCER

Nx Regional lymph nodes cannot be assessed
N0 No regional lymph node metastases
N1 Single ipsilateral node 3 cm or less in diameter
N2a Single ipsilateral node more than 3 cm but not more than 6 cm in diameter
N2b Multiple ipsilateral lymph nodes, none more than 6 cm in diameter
N2c Bilateral or contralateral lymph nodes, none more than 6 cm in diameter
N3 Lymph node more than 6 cm in diameter

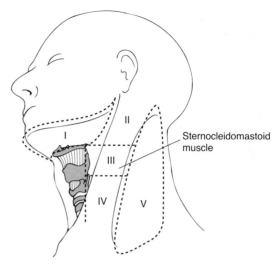

Figure 7.4 – The five 'levels' of lymph nodes in the neck.

Unfortunately, many studies in the past have been carried out on the basis of *clinical staging* which, for the reasons stated below, is often inaccurate. The *pathological* and *radiological staging* also have to be taken into consideration. The pathological staging is not available until after the neck dissection specimen and the primary tumour have been examined by the pathologist. Even then, using the TNM system of staging, two important factors in the prognosis (particularly of oral cancers) have not been considered. These are the site of the primary tumour and its biological activity. It is often a salutary experience to compare the initial clinical staging carried out in the outpatient clinic with the staging following imaging, and then the staging once the specimens have been histologically examined. There is a tendency for surgeons to underestimate the extent of the disease clinically.

The decision on the type of treatment to be employed depends on accurate staging. Unfortunately, there is, at present, a general lack of consensus between surgeons on the best way to treat some head and neck tumours at any particular stage, on the basis of current evidence. How does the staging of the lymph nodes in the neck influence treatment?

The management of malignant lymph nodes in the neck, and the treatment of the N0 neck in particular, remains controversial. The options are surgery, radiotherapy, a combination of the two, or a 'wait and see' policy in the N0 neck. The surgical option involves a neck dissection which is designed to remove various groups of nodes known or thought to be involved in the disease process. The neck is divided into 5 areas or 'levels' for convenience of description (Figure 7.4). These are:

Level I: the nodes in the suprahyoid portion of the anterior triangle of the neck
Level II: the nodes in the upper third of the deep cervical chain
Level III: the nodes in the middle third of the deep cervical chain
Level IV: the nodes in the lower third of the deep cervical chain
Level V: the nodes in the posterior triangle of the neck.

The level II, III and IV nodes are sandwiched between the sternocleidomastoid muscle and the internal jugular vein, between the lower border of the mandible and the clavicle. The chances of any group of nodes being involved vary with the site and size of the primary tumour, as well as its biological activity. For example, the chance of a node in the posterior triangle (level V) being involved is only about 2% for a primary tumour of the anterior two thirds of the tongue. Unfortunately, the spread of tumour to the neck nodes is not entirely predictable, and so the groups of nodes removed in a neck dissection cannot safely be based on probability. Moreover, the disease in the neck is often occult so that the clinical examination is a poor indicator of which nodes are involved. Johnson *et al*[3] have shown that 15% of all patients with oral cancer staged as having an N0 neck will subsequently be found to have lymph node metastases. This is even higher in specific sites such as the tongue, where the figure is nearer 50%.

For these reasons, the operation of choice was the radical neck dissection described by Crile in 1906. In this

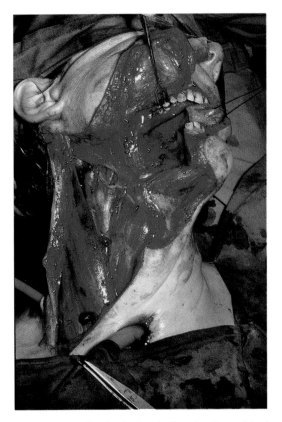

Figure 7.5 – A modified radical neck dissection in combination with a lip split for the removal of a malignant tumour of the posterior floor of the mouth.

procedure all the nodes in levels I–V were removed, along with the accessory nerve, sternocleidomastoid muscle and internal jugular vein. The morbidity was high, particularly with the loss of the accessory nerve. To reduce this morbidity, a more conservative modified radical neck dissection (Figure 7.5) was developed to remove all the nodes in levels I–V but to keep one or more of the major structures, usually the accessory nerve. In such a modified radical neck dissection, the only structures removed might be all the lymph nodes in levels I–V along with the fat and connective tissue enclosing them. The operation is technically more difficult and there is a greater chance of leaving residual disease, particularly if there is extracapsular spread of tumour from the node.

The trend towards selective neck dissection in head and neck cancer

For many years, surgeons have yearned for the time when the pre-operative assessment of the lymph nodes

would be so accurate that only the involved nodes or groups of nodes would require removal. Such an operation is known as a selective neck dissection, as only some of the five levels of nodes are removed. This approach also became increasingly attractive as, with the development of free tissue transfer, it was necessary to enter the neck to identify blood vessels such as the facial artery and internal jugular vein for the purpose of anastomosing the vessels of the donor flap. It was, therefore, a relatively simple matter to extend the dissection to remove the nodes at levels I–III, with virtually no increase in morbidity. This type of selective neck dissection became popular as a supra-omohyoid neck dissection to stage the N0 neck. Nevertheless, the indications for the various selective neck dissections which have been described remain controversial, mainly because of the risk of leaving behind nodes containing tumour. Clearly, this risk would be reduced if a reliable method existed for finding out pre-operatively which nodes contained tumour. In other words, accurate pre-operative imaging of the neck nodes, to show exactly which nodes contained tumour, would allow the surgeon to safely clear the disease from the neck with a quicker operation and less morbidity. The challenge for the future, however, is to find a way of pre-operatively demonstrating micrometastases in a node.

FACTORS WHICH MAY INFLUENCE THE TYPE OF NECK DISSECTION CARRIED OUT FOR HEAD AND NECK CANCER

Size and site of the primary tumour
Thickness of the primary tumour
Histological markers of tumour activity
Size of the neck nodes
Site of the neck nodes (levels I–V)
Presence of tumour in the node
Radiological evidence of extracapsular spread of tumour
Fixed lymph nodes on palpation
Bilateral lymph nodes
Pre-operative radiotherapy
Clinical staging of the tumour
Radiological staging of the tumour
Type of reconstruction to be employed
General health of the patient

It is not the size of the node which contains tumour which is so important, but whether tumour has burst out of the node into the surrounding tissues. The original idea that extranodal spread only occurred in large fixed nodes has been discredited: extranodal spread may occur in a substantial proportion of small nodes. It is, however, true that the greater the size of the node, the greater the chance of extranodal spread: 75% of nodes greater than 3 cm in diameter show extranodal spread. In one study, the 3-year survival rate in patients with positive nodes without extracapsular spread was 52%. In the group with extracapsular spread the 3-year survival dropped to 28% (Figure 7.6).[3] Extracapsular spread to involve the carotid artery usually implies extensive neck invasion which may be unresectable.[4] It is clear, then, that the surgeon not only wishes to know which nodes are involved and at what level, but also whether there has been extracapsular spread of tumour from the node.

> **INFORMATION A SURGEON IDEALLY WANTS TO KNOW ABOUT LYMPH NODES IN THE NECK BEFORE PLANNING TREATMENT**
> Number and size of nodes
> Which nodes are malignant?
> Unilateral or bilateral?
> Level of the nodes (I–V)
> Extracapsular spread of tumour?
> Invasion of adjacent structures?

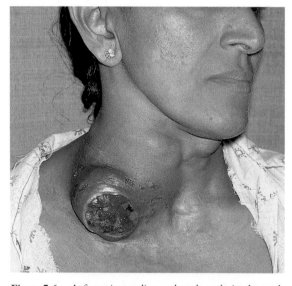

Figure 7.6 – A fungating malignant lymph node in the neck. Recurrent disease in the neck has a very poor prognosis.

The accuracy of clinical assessment of the neck nodes

Surgeons, in general, would like to believe that their clinical diagnosis of neck lumps is accurate, yet the evidence is that their clinical assessment of neck lumps is poor. This is particularly true in the assessment of the neck nodes in cases of head and neck cancer. It is sometimes held that an experienced surgeon can detect a lymph node as small as 0.5 cm if it is superficial, and perhaps a 1 cm node in deeper areas. However, this may prove to be optimistic. Hajek et al,[5] quoting the paper by Sako et al,[6] believe that metastatic lymph nodes less than 12 mm in diameter tend to be missed by clinical examination. Nodes of 12–15 mm size can be palpated only if they are in a superficial position. Those nodes larger than 15 mm in diameter are usually detected by palpation.[5] Clinicians are also usually unable to tell whether the lump is a solitary node or multiple confluent nodes.[6]

Even if the surgeon is able to detect the lymph node, he cannot reliably tell whether the node is 'reactive' or contains tumour. Furthermore, he is unable to detect extranodal spread of tumour or the presence of micrometastases. This difficulty in staging the neck nodes clinically has resulted in studies which attempt to determine which imaging modality, or combination of modalities, gives the most accurate picture of the extent of disease in the neck. In a series of 132 patients, Van den Brekel et al[7] showed that ultrasound in combination with ultrasound-guided aspiration cytology was superior to MRI, CT and ultrasound alone. All imaging techniques were significantly better than palpation. Some controversy still surrounds this issue as the paper of Byers et al[8] concluded that the use of CT and ultrasound was no better than clinical examination in determining the presence or absence of metastatic nodes. Analysis shows, however, that of the 91 patients in the study, only 39 patients had both ultrasound and CT. The scans were performed by sonographers, not radiologists. The comparison and the subsequent conclusion of the authors is therefore questionable. They considered that all patients with a T2–T4 tongue carcinoma should have a neck dissection, and that those in whom the staging was only T1N0 should still have a neck dissection if the depth of muscle invasion was greater than 4 mm, if the tumour was poorly differentiated, or if there was a double DNA–aneuploid tumour.

The criteria on which any diagnostic test is judged are those of specificity and sensitivity. Ideally, the sensitivity should be 100% so that all those patients who require treatment receive it. Similarly, a specificity of 100% would ensure that all patients who do not have disease in the neck will not be subjected to a neck dissection when it is not required. In other words, there would be no false positives or false negatives. In reality, of course, this is unlikely ever to be achieved but it is what a surgeon would like in the ideal world.

THE SURGEON'S VIEW OF THE 'IDEAL' PRE-OPERATIVE INVESTIGATION FOR A NECK LUMP
Absolute specificity
Absolute sensitivity
Accurate tissue diagnosis
Minimally invasive
Cheap

How accurate is the clinical assessment of a neck node by a clinician? It has been shown that even an experienced clinician's examination of the neck is unreliable when assessing lymph nodes. Baatenburg and his colleagues[9] reviewed the literature and concluded that palpation of the neck has a false positive rate of between 15% and 65% (most authors quote about 25%), and a false negative rate of between 10% and 15%. A number of studies reported elsewhere in this book have compared these results with the specificity and sensitivity of MRI, CT and ultrasound (with or without fine-needle aspiration cytology). The results show that some types of imaging significantly help the surgeon to visualise more clearly the extent and pattern of the disease in the neck. According to the criteria necessary to justify a radiological investigation, it would then be necessary to demonstrate that the information would influence the management decisions of the surgeon.

Hajek et al[5] showed that ultrasound examination changed the planned operation in 55% of cases (in 41% a more radical operation was undertaken, and in 14% ultrasound showed that the tumour was inoperable). In 43 patients (58%), ultrasound revealed extra, unknown or clinically unsuspected findings. Evidence of tumour infiltration of the carotid arteries changed the operative course remarkably.

More accurate staging of the neck may thus alter the surgical plan in a number of ways. The neck dissection may be more radical than is indicated by clinical examination. A bilateral rather than a unilateral neck dissec-

tion might be necessary, or a selective neck dissection to clear different levels of nodes may be carried out.

Imaging also has an important part to play in the postoperative phase. If a clinical recurrence is suspected many months after the resection, it may be difficult for the radiologist to differentiate between changes due to previous surgery and radiotherapy and changes due to recurrent tumour. It is therefore an advantage to have repeat imaging performed relatively soon after the completion of treatment, so that the radiologist has a baseline with which to compare later images taken for a suspected recurrence.

Does improved imaging result in a better outcome for the patient?

Although modern imaging techniques do enable the surgeon to tailor treatment more effectively, the question remains 'Is there evidence to show that this has improved the outcome for the patient?'. Common sense dictates that patients can only benefit from more informed treatment planning. In head and neck cancer, however, the evidence is sparse. There appears to have been little improvement over the last 35 years in the overall 5-year survival rate in squamous cell carcinoma of the upper aerodigestive tract, which remains at about 40%. Assessment of outcome involves not only crude mortality data but quality of life data which are more difficult to collect. Such data are beginning to emerge and it may prove possible to show that better imaging does improve the quality of survival in head and neck cancer patients, and possibly survival rates as well.

In an ideal world, a surgeon operating on a lump would like to know exactly what it is and where it is before he operates. In this way it should be possible to obtain the best outcome for the patient with the least morbidity. The hope is that the further development of imaging techniques may enable this to become a reality.

References

1. Shah JP. Cervical lymph node metastasis. Diagnostic, therapeutic and prognostic implications. *Oncology* 1990; **4(10):** 61–69.

2. Snow GB, Patel P, Leemans CR, Tiwari R. Management of cervical lymph nodes in patients with head and neck cancer. *Eur Arch Otorhinolaryngol* 1992; **249:** 187–194.

3. Johnson JT, Barnes EL, Myers EN. The extracapsular spread of tumours in cervical node metastasis. *Arch Otolaryngol* 1981; **107:** 725.

4. Ogura JH, Biller HF. Head and neck – surgical management. *JAMA* 1972; **221:** 77–79.

5. Hajek PC, Salomonowitz E, Turk R, Tscholakoff D, Kumpan W, Czembirek H. Lymph nodes of the neck: evaluation with US. *Radiology* 1986; **158:** 739–742.

6. Sako K, Pradier RN, Marchetta FC, Pickren JW. Fallibility of palpation in the diagnosis of metastases to cervical nodes. *Surg Gyn Obstet* 1964; **118:** 989–990.

7. Van den Brekel MWM, Castelijns JA, Stel HV, Golding RP, Meyer CJL, Snow GB. Modern imaging techniques and ultrasound-guided aspiration cytology for the assessment of neck node metastases: a prospective comparative study. *Eur Arch Otorhinolaryngol* 1993; **250:** 11–17.

8. Byers RM, El-Naggar AK, Lee YY *et al.* Can we detect or predict the presence of occult nodal metastases in patients with squamous carcinoma of the oral tongue? *Head Neck* 1998; **20:** 138–144.

9. Baatenburg de Jong RJ, Rongen RJ, Lameris JS, Harthoorn M, Verwoerd CDA, Knegt P. Metastatic neck disease: palpation vs ultrasound examination. *Arch Otolaryngol Head Neck Surg* 1989; **115:** 689–690.

8

FINE-NEEDLE ASPIRATION OR CORE BIOPSY?

NJA Cozens, L Berman

Fine-needle aspiration

Core biopsy

Introduction

Once started on the learning curve for head and neck ultrasound, the radiologist will rapidly approach the next hurdle – namely, how best to acquire a tissue diagnosis? Ultrasound lends itself to biopsy techniques in the neck, being far superior to magnetic resonance imaging (MRI) and computed tomography (CT) in this respect.

Which technique should be the first choice of the radiologist – fine-needle aspiration (FNA) or core biopsy? The straight answer is that FNA should be the initial choice in the majority of cases; the answer will be obtained in 80% of cases provided there is local cytological expertise. But, if FNA is so successful, what is the role for core biopsy? Core biopsy has two roles to play: to give an answer when the cytologist cannot, and to give a tissue diagnosis which may obviate the need for an open biopsy. Where histological expertise allows, oncologists may opt to treat lymphoma diagnosed and typed by a core biopsy rather than open biopsy. The benefit to the patient and clinician alike in speed of diagnosis and reduced morbidity is obvious.

Children are always a special case in radiology, and biopsy techniques are no exception. Core biopsy techniques are now so refined that biopsy is now possible in children without the use of sedation. This practice is not universal, but it is a development that should not be ignored.

The choice between core biopsy and FNA will always be governed by local factors and influences. Allowing for these influences, the evidence produced in this chapter should allow the radiologist to make an informed decision as to the choice of biopsy technique.

Fine-needle aspiration

N J A Cozens

Background

Fine-needle aspiration (FNA) has had a long history. Its incorporation into daily clinical practice stems from the 1950s, with the development of an FNA clinic at the Cancer Centre of the Karolinska Hospital in Stockholm, where pathologists took and interpreted the specimens. Initially, clinicians also took FNAs and sent them to the clinic for diagnosis but this practice was soon discouraged because of the poor quality of samples.[1] Many clinicians still undertake 'blind' FNA of head and neck lesions; the specimens obtained are poor compared to those obtained with ultrasound guidance.

Suitability of ultrasound guidance

The combination of ultrasound assessment and guidance for FNA in head and neck lesions maximises the quality of specimens and thus the information available to the patient and clinician to optimise patient care. Real-time ultrasound guidance is ideally suited for FNA in this area of the body as it is accurate, inexpensive, well tolerated and quick.[2,3] The proximity to the skin surface of these superficial structures suits ultrasound guidance perfectly. Ultrasound-guided FNA can therefore be more accurate than CT, MRI or ultrasound alone in determining pathological involvement of tissues.[4–8]

Advantages and disadvantages of fine-needle aspiration

Advantages of FNA include the minimal cost and number of materials required for obtaining a specimen, the relatively inexpensive cytopathology laboratory processing costs and speed of both obtaining a specimen and the cytological diagnosis. The potential morbidity for the patient is also very small, with minor discomfort during the procedure and occasional bruising or rarely a small post-procedure haematoma.[9]

The disadvantages can all be considered as dependent on the operator. The adequacy of the sample depends upon the expertise of the person performing the FNA; this is considered below. The usefulness of the cytological report depends upon several factors. The accuracy of the reports is critical: an unacceptable false positive or, in particular, false negative rate can negate any potential benefit of FNA. The percentage of equivocal reports from adequate samples also affects the usefulness of FNA and must be minimised. Accurate cytological interpretation of the sample depends upon its being accompanied by accurate clinical information, a factor frequently overlooked by those obtaining the samples. The interrelated factors above make appropriate cytopathological expertise[10] a prerequisite for provision of a useful FNA service. This expertise is becoming more widespread but it is often the limiting factor preventing widespread acceptance of FNA.

The specific tissue-related pitfalls relate to the difficulty in making a definitive diagnosis in some specific lesions, as in subgrouping of lymphoma,[11] which depends upon the histological architecture of lymph nodes.

POTENTIAL ADVANTAGES AND DISADVANTAGES OF FNA
Advantages
Minimal materials
Inexpensive
Speed
Minimal morbidity

Disadvantages
Sample adequacy
False positive/false negative/equivocal aspirates
Dependence on cytopathology expertise
Specific tissue-related potential pitfalls

Who should perform fine-needle aspiration?

There are many alternative strategies for performing FNA. The guiding factors are local circumstances, attitudes and availability of appropriate personnel. Various possibilities are considered below.

INDIVIDUALS

Clinician

Many clinicians perform FNAs in the outpatient clinic, if lesions are palpable. The immediacy of this type of FNA makes it quick and convenient for the patient. However clinicians consistently provide the worst samples, with the highest inadequate specimen rate[12] (particularly if they only perform FNA occasionally) and, more significantly, the highest false negative rate for malignant lesions.

Pathologist

There are several advantages in pathologists performing FNAs:

- the ability to maintain competency by a single aspirator regularly performing FNAs in greater numbers than an individual clinician

- availability of enhanced clinical information, as compared to the 'lump in neck – FNA' frequently present on pathology request forms from clinician aspirators

- the ability to make direct smears and assess specimen adequacy at the bedside or in the clinic.

Radiologist

The major advantage is assessment of the neck with ultrasound, enabling accurate, relevant, representative samples of palpable and impalpable lesions to be obtained while avoiding adjacent normal tissues. Normal anatomical variants are also readily identified and confirmed.[13] As patients can be referred by many different clinicians, expertise is concentrated,[12] ensuring that a high level of competence in performing FNA can be achieved and maintained.

TEAM APPROACH

- Clinician/cytology technician
- Clinician/cytopathologist
- Cytopathologist/cytology technician
- Radiologist/cytology technician
- Radiologist/cytopathologist.

The possible combinations listed above depend upon local expertise and availability. Any of these combinations has the potential to be better than any of the individuals separately, but they are more expensive and potentially less versatile.

In day-to-day working practice the decision whether to perform an FNA is made at the time of the ultrasound examination. The immediacy of this decision precludes the attendance of a cytopathologist or cytology technician in most instances. It is therefore incumbent on the radiologist and attending radiographers/nurses to be trained in slide preparation techniques. This arrangement should result in adequate sampling in 80–85% of cases. In those cases where the initial FNA is inadequate, however, a repeat FNA should be performed in the presence of a cytology technician or cytopathologist.

The combination best able to optimise specimen acquisition, processing and assessment is that of radiologist and cytopathologist. The factors affecting this model are presented below.

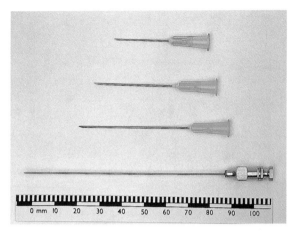

Figure 8.1 – Needles for FNA. In ascending order: 22 G 90 mm spinal needle, 21 G 50 and 40 mm, and 23 G 25 mm 'Microlance 3' needles.

Equipment required for fine-needle aspiration

Apart from access to a high quality ultrasound machine with a high resolution, high frequency (e.g. 5–10 MHz) transducer, relatively little equipment is required for FNA. A further advantage is that the equipment used is both inexpensive and readily available. If a choice of linear transducers of appropriate frequency is available, the transducer with the smallest footprint is optimal. This is particularly relevant for lesions in the head and neck. The superficial position of the structures, combined with high frequency transducers, obviates the need to consider using a biopsy guide with ultrasound-guided methods of FNA.

NEEDLES

A variety of needles are available for FNA (Figure 8.1). The most suitable needle for almost all aspiration within the head and neck is a standard 21 gauge needle (Microlance 3, Becton Dickinson). Although a 23 gauge provides adequate cytological specimens, it is only available in 25 mm or 30 mm lengths, which can limit the accessibility of lesions. This is particularly relevant when using the angled technique relative to the transducer. The use of a 21 gauge needle does not significantly increase side effects, and it is available in both 40 mm and 50 mm lengths (which have a measured 37 mm and 50 mm of needle shaft respectively). In

practice, the longer 50 mm needle proves more versatile for targeting and aspirating lesions, allowing access at all angles and depths within the head and neck.

A needle with an internal stylet may occasionally be useful to prevent aspiration of tissue fragments from the needle track before reaching the lesion. A standard 9 cm long, 22 gauge spinal needle proves adequate for this, although the extra length and flexibility make it slightly more difficult to manoeuvre accurately.

The 23 gauge venesection type needle described above can occasionally be useful to obtain a sample from a small, very superficial or mobile nodule which has proved impossible to puncture with the standard 21 gauge needle.

SYRINGES/EXTENSION TUBING

When suction aspiration is required, a 10 or 20 ml syringe is attached to a flexible fine bore connecting tube (Figure 8.2). The optimal length is between 20 and 50 cm to allow manoeuvrability without the need to exert excessive suction pressure to overcome the internal resistance of a longer tube. The needle is attached to the other end of the tubing prior to needle placement within the patient.

SYRINGE HOLDER

Syringe holders are available to facilitate aspiration as a single-handed procedure. In practice these are too bulky and cumbersome for many lesions in the head

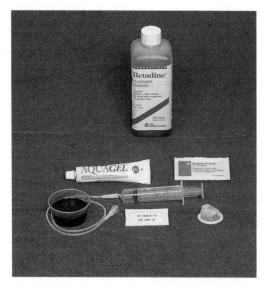

Figure 8.2 – Miscellaneous equipment for FNA. Syringe, extension tubing (50 cm), Betadine (Seton Healthcare Group, PLC) antiseptic solution with gallipot container, alcohol swab, lubricating jelly (Aquagel, Adams Healthcare) and a Durex Dry® condom.

and neck, reducing the accuracy of needle placement. Capillary technique or the use of an assistant to provide negative pressure via the syringe and extension tubing is preferred.

STERILITY

Many articles in the FNA literature make no mention of sterility or prevention of cross-contamination between patients via the ultrasound transducer. The most frequently quoted method of equipment sterilisation between patients is wiping the transducer with an alcohol-based swab. There is evidence that this method may not remove traces of blood between patients. Also, some manufacturers contraindicate alcohol swabs as they potentially damage transducers. The use of a condom, transducer cover or cling film has therefore been advocated. A condom often proves ideal, being sterile, individually packed, and cheaper than the specialised transducer covers available. A nonlubricated condom such as Durex Dry® (or Durex Ultrasound Probe Cover®) prevents unwanted transducer slipperiness that can impair accuracy of needle placement (Figure 8.2).

Sterile aqueous jelly, aqueous iodine solution, chlorhexidine or alcohol solution can all act as coupling agents between the skin and the condom-covered transducer.

LOCAL ANAESTHETIC

Local anaesthesia is rarely required; the injection of lignocaine is usually more painful than the FNA itself. The exception is in children, where the application of topical local anaesthetic cream one hour before the FNA is beneficial.

CYTOSPIN FLUID

If it is not possible to have direct slide preparations made immediately by a pathologist or cytopathology technician at the time the FNA is taken, it is best to place the specimen into a transport medium for later slide preparation in the laboratory, e.g. Cytospin collection fluid (Shandon, UK) containing ethanol, carbowax and isopropyl alcohol. Slides can thus be obtained in the pathology laboratory that are of consistently higher quality than those prepared by us as radiologists. The cells are retrieved by centrifuge, and red blood cells are lysed before specimen preparation. This technique will not work for suspected lipomas.

SLIDES/1% AQUEOUS TOLUIDINE BLUE/ALCOHOL/ BENCH MICROSCOPE

These are the tools of the pathologist or cytology technician for immediate assessment of adequacy of samples.

INCONTINENCE SHEETS

Incontinence sheets are essential equipment for the pathologist! Toluidine blue stains everything it contacts, including ultrasound department work surfaces. Incontinence sheets to protect the departmental work surfaces will prove invaluable!

Practical fine-needle aspiration techniques

1 Perform an initial comprehensive neck ultrasound examination.
2 Is FNA required?
3 Which site/s are appropriate?
4 The choice of node or other site/s should be influenced by its potential impact on management.

Masses within the head and neck, and their nature, are examined in detail in other chapters of this book. Any lesion that is suspicious may be subjected to FNA to complement the ultrasound assessment.[15,16] The practical aspects of FNA are described in detail below.

Fine-needle aspiration is well tolerated by almost all patients. Explanation of the procedure should include an honest appraisal of the relatively mild and transient discomfort felt during the FNA. The patient must be instructed to stay still, and not to swallow if the thyroid is targeted. Local anaesthetic is almost never required; the most apprehensive of patients can be reassured and calmed by having an assistant's hand to hold during the procedure.

The techniques for FNA vary between individuals and institutions – there is no single 'correct' way of performing an FNA. The following observations are therefore not prescriptive, but constitute a personal adaptation of various techniques which currently provide adequate material for cytological assessment in more than 95% of head and neck masses. The immediate assessment of each FNA pass has enabled the evolution of these techniques, facilitated by interaction between radiologist and cytopathologist to minimise the number of needle passes required and maximise diagnostic yield.

PATIENT POSITION

The patient's position is dictated by the location of the target organ, node or mass. The patient is usually supine, with neck extended and head rotated as necessary to optimise access.

PATIENT AND TRANSDUCER PREPARATION

Many centres choose to use a simple skin disinfection procedure with an alcohol based swab, and no cover on the transducer. An alternative, potentially safer technique is to prepare the skin with an alcohol based swab, then use a sterile disposable condom as a transducer cover. The addition of a small amount of aqueous jelly inside the condom ensures optimal transducer contact. The coupling medium between condom and patient can be either sterile aqueous jelly or aqueous 'skin preparation' antiseptic such as 10% povidone–iodine solution. The latter preparation prevents blood-borne infective agents being transmitted from patient to patient (a theoretical possibility).

SUCTION ASPIRATION

This is the most commonly used technique for obtaining FNA samples. Approximately 2 ml of air is introduced into the syringe before aspiration, facilitating optimal specimen retrieval as it is then possible to expel the contents of the needle lumen and hub immediately, rather than sucking them into the syringe prior to expulsion. Syringe holders are too bulky and insensitive for FNA in the head and neck.

Although it is technically possible to attach a needle directly to a syringe and single-handedly target the lesion with this combination, withdrawing the syringe plunger when the needle is within the lesion reduces manoeuvrability. By introducing a 20–50 cm length of extension tubing between the needle and syringe, it is possible to have an assistant provide the negative suction pressure without interfering with needle placement. The optimal technique for suction aspiration is to have an assistant provide approximately 5 ml of suction while the needle is within the lesion and release suction prior to withdrawal from the lesion. This allows the radiologist to manipulate the transducer and needle most accurately to obtain the best needle placement. The aspiration should be terminated if blood is seen entering the connecting tubing as this contaminates the specimen without increasing the cellular specimen yield. Once the needle is removed, the patient is asked to press firmly on a sterile swab placed over the puncture site.

CAPILLARY CONCEPT – ADVANTAGES

An alternative strategy, which is rarely advocated in the radiological literature but has become our technique of first choice with most head and neck lesions, is to utilise a capillary technique for obtaining samples.[1,17–23]

The principle is that the negative pressure applied in the suction technique above plays a relatively minor role compared to the cutting or scraping action of the sharp bevelled needle within the tissue. The additional cytological observation that the capillary pressure alone is sufficient to retain the cells within the lumen of a fine bore (25–21 G) needle adds objective evidence to the theory that suction may be superfluous (Figure 8.3).

The advantages are particularly important in head and neck FNA. Improved sensitivity and ability to manipulate the needle results from holding the needle hub between forefinger and thumb without the relatively cumbersome syringe or tubing connected. Contamination with blood during sampling is significantly reduced using the capillary method; this is particularly advantageous in the thyroid. The cell yield may also be reduced, but this does not adversely affect the specimen quality or the ability to obtain diagnostic FNA samples in this region of the body. A further practical advantage is that it is often possible to access the lesion, obtain the sample and withdraw the needle more rapidly with the capillary technique than with suction aspiration. This is advantageous in particularly anxious or less co-operative patients, especially in

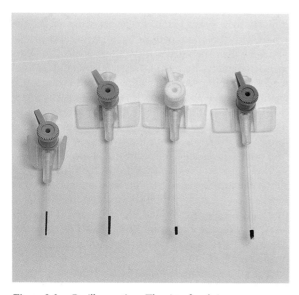

Figure 8.3 – Capillary action. The tip of each intravenous cannula was dipped into iodine solution and held vertically. The difference between the lengths of cannula filled illustrates that the capillary action is inversely proportional to the diameter of the tube lumen. Size ranges from 22 G (0.8 mm, blue cap) to 14 G (2.0 mm brown cap).

potentially mobile tissue such as the thyroid. The box below summarises personal experience, suggesting sites that may be appropriate for either suction or capillary action aspirates. It may be appropriate to attempt to obtain aspirates by both techniques in many cases, particularly if immediate specimen evaluation is not available.

FNA TECHNIQUES

Capillary technique
Thyroid
Lymph nodes
Salivary gland
Vascular lesions on colour Doppler

Suction techniques
Fibrotic lymph nodes (post therapy)
Cystic lesions
?Lipoma
Any lesion in which two initial capillary
aspirates yield no sample
?Abscess

NEEDLE ROTATION/MICROCORES

The role played by rotation of the needle whilst the sample is being taken is another practical observation that is only occasionally mentioned in the radiological literature. Rotation of the sharp, bevelled needle tip often produces tiny cores within the lumen of the needle – 'microcores' – which are also frequently evident on cytological preparations if smeared directly onto microscope slides.

The analogy between attempting to push a drill bit through the softest pine by hand and comparing the hole and wood fragments produced with a hole drilled by the same bit in a slowly rotating hand drill should convince radiologists to adopt rotation during FNA procurement (Figure 8.4).

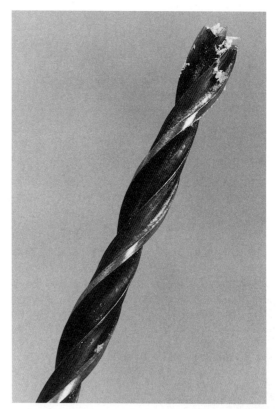

Figure 8.4 – Needle rotation. A drill bit analogy emphasises the importance of needle rotation during FNA.

SAMPLING SITE

The appropriate site or lesion for FNA can be predicted from features covered in other chapters. It is also important to obtain samples from multiple sites on occasion, particularly from any suspected primary carcinoma with suspicious associated lymph nodes.

The periphery of a lesion is frequently the most informative site for FNA. This is particularly crucial if there is any central necrosis. Occasionally, cystic or necrotic metastatic lymph nodes can have their contents aspirated by a single initial suction needle pass, followed by a second aspirate from the collapsed wall, which is more likely to yield diagnostic viable tumour cells if these are present.

NUMBER OF PASSES

The number of passes required is easy to determine if the radiologist is in the privileged position of having immediate cytological assessment available. This is the ideal situation, but for many institutions it cannot often be achieved. The decision then depends mainly upon local circumstances: the more experienced the radiologist and cytopathologist, the fewer the passes required. With immediate cytological assessment it is feasible to obtain good specimens with a single needle pass in over 80% of patients.

If Cytospin transport medium is used it is sometimes possible to guess whether the sample is likely to be satisfactory by gently swirling the fluid after the specimen has been expelled into it, and looking for obvious tissue fragments or 'microcores' (Figure 8.5). This is most likely to be feasible after a capillary FNA when there is minimal blood contamination to obscure the fluid.

ANGLED VERSUS VERTICAL APPROACH

The method of approach relative to the transducer is determined by personal preference and accessibility to each potential FNA site. Many radiologists routinely use a vertical approach, lining up the centre of the linear transducer with the target and introducing the needle adjacent to the middle of the long axis of the transducer, angling the needle vertically downwards and slightly towards the transducer. Although the needle tip can be visualised throughout the FNA, one does not see the entire length of the needle with this approach. It is consistently reproducible, and is sometimes the only possible safe trajectory available to avoid traversing the trachea, carotid artery, etc. It can, however, be difficult to sample selectively the periphery of the lesion, particularly its superficial aspects (Figure 8.6).

The alternative is to approach the lesion from an angle (usually between 20 and 60 degrees), inserting the needle adjacent to the middle of the short axis of the transducer. Although this can be more difficult to learn initially, the advantage is clear visualisation of the whole shaft of the needle throughout the FNA (Figure 8.7). This is most pertinent when trying to aspirate small or mobile lesions. It also provides an alternative route to lesions inaccessible to direct vertical sampling.

The two approaches are therefore complementary. Each radiologist will become more comfortable per-

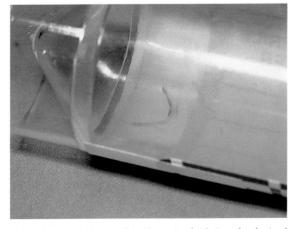

Figure 8.5 – A 'microcore' in Cytospin fluid. Sample obtained with capillary technique and a 21 G needle.

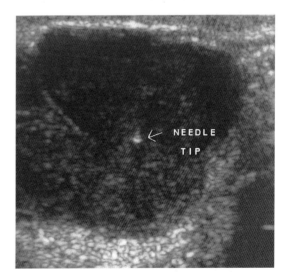

Figure 8.6 – Vertical needle approach. The tiny echogenic focus within this pleomorphic salivary gland adenoma is the needle tip during FNA.

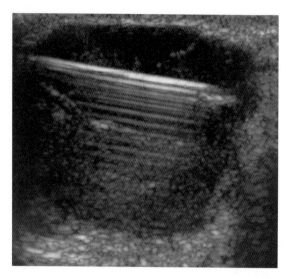

Figure 8.7 – Angled needle approach. The whole shaft and even the bevelled tip of the same 21 G needle is seen within the same pleomorphic salivary gland adenoma as in Figure 8.6.

forming most FNAs with one approach, but should be able to use the alternative when it is necessary.

SPECIMEN HANDLING

The specimen is likely to be prepared most expertly by either a cytopathologist or cytology technician. If immediate preparation and assessment is not available in the ultrasound department, transport in Cytospin fluid is usually the best method.

CYTOLOGY REPORT REVIEW

Constant review of our performance is crucial to achieve and maintain high standards of clinically useful FNAs. It is essential that the radiologist receives a copy of the cytology report on every FNA carried out. Histological and clinical review is also essential to detect any false negative or false positive results.

Acknowledgement

The author would like to thank Dr Ivan Robinson for his pivotal role in the development of our combined ultrasound-guided cytology clinic. His cytological expertise has not only facilitated clinically crucial decisions to be taken pre-operatively, but also enabled the incorporation of techniques adopted from cytopathological practice to enhance specimen acquisition.

Core biopsy

L Berman

Introduction

Fine-needle aspiration (FNA) of head and neck masses is an established safe technique, particularly in the thyroid gland where it provides material for cytological diagnosis. Ultrasound guidance improves the accuracy of FNA[24–27] and is particularly helpful when lesions are impalpable or when 'blind' unguided aspiration has failed to provide adequate material.[28,29]

Ultrasound-guided core biopsies are easily performed as outpatient procedures but do require a little more time than FNA.[30,31] Core biopsy needles are undoubtedly more costly than any of the currently used FNA needles, but the biopsy needle represents a small fraction of the total cost of the procedure. Furthermore, the success of the technique is not enhanced by the presence of a pathologist at the bedside to process the specimen, as it is usually obvious from the naked eye examination that adequate tissue has been obtained.

The author's intention is to explore where the technique sits with existing practice, which for the most part relies on FNA or surgical resection, usually omitting what could be considered to be the intermediate stage of tissue core biopsy.

Despite the widespread adoption of core biopsy in other sites such as the breast, and given the impact that a core biopsy service can make on surgical and oncological practice, it is surprising that there are few reports of the technique being used in the head and neck.[30–32]

Indications and patient selection

Core biopsy should be considered as complementary to, rather than as a rival of, FNA. It is unwise to be proscriptive about the indications for the technique, as the readiness and need for a department to undertake this procedure depend on factors such as the patient population, referral pattern, and availability of an accurate cytological service. An important issue is the ability of pathologists to make a definitive diagnosis, e.g. in cases of lymphoma, on the basis of tissue obtained from a core rather than the entire lymph node. Equally important is the confidence of the referring clinician in that diagnosis prior to commencing therapy. The indications will also depend on the organ of origin, the suspected diagnosis, the presence of a known malignancy, and whether the procedure will obviate the need for further surgery.

Leaving aside the exact details of disease process, there are two broad clinical indications: firstly, where it is the aim of the clinician to avoid an open surgical procedure by obtaining tissue by percutaneous biopsy; and, secondly, where although surgery is anticipated as part of curative therapy, it may be modified depending on the histological findings.

ADVANTAGES OF CORE BIOPSY
Inexpensive
Relatively atraumatic
May obviate the need for open biopsy
Higher diagnostic yield

Needle design

Automated 'one-handed' core biopsy needles have gained wide acceptance in imaging departments, both for the sampling of large target organs such as the liver, as well as for smaller lesions such as those of the breast, which require extremely accurate guidance. The cutting action of these spring-loaded devices varies. Some require the cutting notch to be positioned proximal to the biopsy site, as both the inner stylet and the outer cutting blade jump forward on triggering. With small lesions, the needle would actually have to be outside the lesion before triggering. This spring-loaded action of the inner stylet may be advantageous when biopsying extremely dense lesions in the breast but these 'advancing' needles would not be acceptable in the head and neck because of the risk of damage to adjacent vulnerable structures such as the major neck vessels, trachea or brachial plexus.

Several makes of disposable needle are available in which the inner stylet with its cutting notch are manually advanced into the lesion. Very few head and neck lesions are sufficiently dense or scirrhous to prevent the gentle, precise, controlled advancement of the cutting notch into an optimal position for biopsy. On triggering, only the cutting blade advances over the stylet. The specimen notch, which is invariably demonstrated on the ultrasound localisation, can be positioned exactly at the intended biopsy site. Triggering is achieved by further pressure with the thumb on the handle of the central stylet. As there is no forward

motion of the entire needle, this design is safer for use within the neck (Figure 8.8).

To this end, we have collaborated with the makers of one disposable needle (Temno, Bauer Medical Inc., FL, USA) to produce a design that we find safer for neck core biopsies (Figure 8.9). The needle is available in 18 and 16 SWG diameters and in 8 cm and 16 cm lengths. The specimen notch in the stylet is 1.5 cm in length but there are models of needle where a 'variable throw' may be used to obtain specimens of 5 mm, 10 mm or 15 mm. It is helpful if the stylet tip is as sharp as possible. This is particularly important in the thyroid where it may be difficult to penetrate the surrounding fascia with the needle tip.

With modern ultrasound apparatus needle visibility is no longer an issue and so roughened or grooved stylet tips are of no particular advantage.

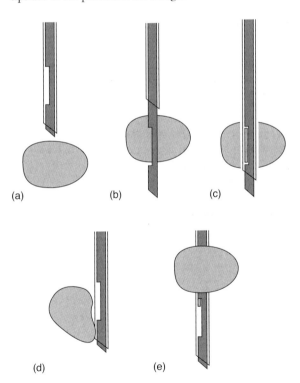

(a)   (b)   (c)

(d)   (e)

Figure 8.8 – (a) The pre-triggering position of an advancing cutting needle. On triggering, the central stylet advances into the lesion (b) followed by the outer blade (c). (d, e) The potential pitfalls of advancing needles. The stylet of a 'non-advancing' cutting needle is manually advanced (with the central stylet extended) into the intended biopsy site (b). On triggering, only the outer blade advances over the stylet. There is no risk of damaging adjacent structures or of 'deflecting' the lesion.

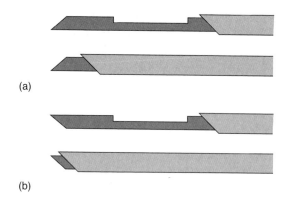

(a)

(b)

Figure 8.9 – Differences in needle tip design. The needle illustrated in (b) is preferred to the conventional needle design shown in (a) as there is a shorter length of the stylet projecting beyond the specimen notch and outer blade, reducing the risk of damaging adjacent structures.

General hints and pitfalls

This description is confined to those hints and pitfalls that are specific to head and neck cutting needle biopsies.

The technique will vary according to the site and organ of origin of the lesion. We use 16 SWG needles for all except the smallest lymph nodes or thyroid nodules, where we would use an 18 SWG needle. In all cases a 1.5 cm cutting notch is used; if the diameter of lesion is much smaller than 1.5 cm, we inform the pathologists to expect to find the lesion sandwiched between normal adjacent tissue. The need for adequate communication with both clinician and pathologist cannot be overstated. All of our core biopsies are examined by a single pathologist and this may explain the success of the technique at our institute, particularly in the setting of lymphoma.

Of equal importance is the need for adequate communication with the patient. Many of the patients are biopsied at their first visit to the ultrasound department. In addition to an explanation by the referring clinician, they are sent a form giving them details of what to expect if a biopsy is undertaken. A contact telephone number is supplied if they wish to enquire about any aspect of the procedure. If the patient is on anticoagulation therapy we are prepared to undertake lymph node biopsy using an 18 SWG needle only. As mild post-biopsy bleeding is usually more noticeable with thyroid lesions, we regard anticoagulation as an absolute contraindication to outpatient thyroid core biopsies.

Practical technique

A comprehensive ultrasound examination is performed, including colour Doppler studies. The Doppler study is not undertaken out of mere curiosity. A colour flow Doppler study defines internal vascularity and avoids the pitfall of dismissing a lesion as a cyst. In the thyroid, the presence of vessels within a mural soft tissue component to a cyst may distinguish it from adherent residual mural thrombus resulting from a bleed into a cyst.

Following the initial study and choice of approach, the couch or ultrasound machine is moved so that the operator can easily sight across the patient towards the ultrasound monitor. The hand–eye co-ordination required for the procedure is not helped by having to crane round to view the monitor while the needle is in the patient.

An important point that we learned early in our experience was to rehearse the sound of the needle spring action with the patient *before* attempting the biopsy. By definition, the mechanism is close to the patient's ear. The spring action makes a loud click that could cause the patient to jump while the needle is still within the lesion. At the time of the actual biopsy patients should be warned to anticipate a loud click. After the biopsy the patient applies gentle pressure with a sterile swab while the specimen is examined and transferred to a container. In almost every case the patient is able to leave the department following a brief period of observation and a hot drink. If there is a haematoma or swelling at the biopsy site a repeat ultrasound scan will demonstrate whether there has been a significant bleed.

We use a high frequency linear array transducer of at least 7.5 MHz and perform all biopsies as freehand procedures. We have no personal experience of using a needle guide in this situation. The cutting notch should always be uppermost, i.e. directed towards the transducer. This ensures that the notch, which is easily identified on the image, is accurately positioned within the lesion. In addition, the flat surface of the base of the notch is much more conspicuous on the ultrasound image than the curved surface of the needle.

All our biopsies have been performed in a transverse plane, i.e. with the needle perpendicular to the long axis of the probe. Important structures that one would wish to avoid, such as the carotid artery, are always demonstrated in a transverse image of the neck. This enables the needle tip's relationship to the carotid artery to be continually monitored. When scanning or inserting a needle parallel to the vessels, it is much more difficult to monitor these relationships as the carotid may not be demonstrated in the image that shows the needle within the lesion.

Specific applications

LYMPH NODES

These are usually far easier to biopsy than thyroid or salivary gland lesions. The closed stylet and blade are advanced to the periphery of the lesion. By advancing the central stylet with thumb pressure the cutting notch appears from within the surrounding blade and the needle is triggered once the cutting notch is positioned within the node. Extremely superficial lesions require the needle to be inserted horizontally several centimetres away from the biopsy site as part of the cutting notch and the entire blade would actually be outside the patient prior to triggering if a more vertical approach was used (Figure 8.10).

If there is the slightest chance of a diagnosis of lymphoma, the core should be placed in a dry sterile container and not in formalin. In our series of core biopsies there has been complete classification of lymphomas including definitive immunocytochemical studies in over 85% of our biopsies.

Similarly, if an infective lesion is even a remote possibility, a second core should be obtained and placed in a dry sterile container. All dry specimens should be transferred immediately to the pathology department. A surprising number (8%) of our lymph node biopsies, particularly in apparently well children and young adults, have yielded tuberculosis or atypical mycobacteria. If there is the slightest clinical or sonographic suspicion of a mass being due to mycobacterial infection rather than lymphoma, a second core is obtained for microbiological studies.

In patients with a known primary there is little advantage in carrying out a core biopsy rather than a FNA. FNA is more successful in diagnosing or excluding malignancy in patients with a known head and neck primary.[33–35]

THYROID

There are two indications for core biopsy in the thyroid:

1 when the initial FNA has failed to provide an adequate specimen
2 when the initial cytological analysis was equivocal.

The thyroid is a soft, deformable organ with a surrounding fascia that may be difficult to penetrate with the needle tip. Although colour flow studies frequently demonstrate an alarmingly vascular organ, this is not a contraindication to biopsy.

In many situations it is possible to approach the lesion lateromedially through or close to the sternomastoid and with the stylet tip directed towards the trachea. The same lesion may be approached mediolaterally, avoiding the trachea but with the needle tip directed towards the major neck vessels. Both approaches have their advantages and drawbacks. If the gland is particularly mobile a lateromedial approach will steady it against the trachea during insertion of the needle. Injury to the trachea should not occur if the needle is always manipulated under direct guidance.

In practice, the operator varies the approach according to his or her handedness, the side of the pathology, and the exact site and size of the lesion. It is possible to aim for extremely small mural components of predominantly cystic thyroid lesions, and these are more easily biopsied with an 18 SWG needle (Figure 8.11). Thick-walled cystic lesions are readily biopsied without prior aspiration of the contents by inserting an 18 SWG

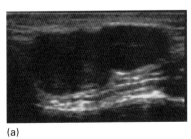 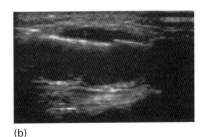 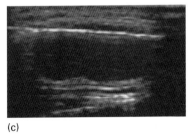

(a) (b) (c)

Figure 8.10 – A superficial node requiring a horizontal subcutaneous approach (a); (b) shows the needle with stylet advanced and the specimen notch demonstrated clearly within the lesion; (c) the needle following triggering.

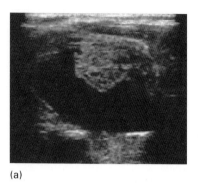 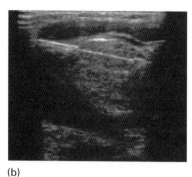 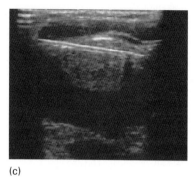

(a)   (b)   (c)

Figure 8.11 – A complex thyroid nodule (a). Biopsy is targeted to the solid element, the specimen notch straddling the mural nodule (b). The needle following triggering (c).

needle tangentially along the wall and avoiding the cystic component.

If a suspicious lymph node is demonstrated in the region of a thyroid nodule, particularly if the nodule is hypo-echoic and the lymph node contains fine scattered calcification, we routinely biopsy both structures.

Thyroid specimens are always transported in formalin.

SALIVARY GLAND

Damage to the facial nerve will be a concern to newcomers to this technique, however the retromandibular vein is an excellent landmark for the facial nerve; it is therefore necessary to identify and avoid the retromandibular vein in all biopsies.

We attempt to insert the needle as superficially as possible, following a horizontal subcutaneous course. The most superficial aspect of the lesion is biopsied. If bilateral pathology is demonstrated we only biopsy one (the easier) side, making the admittedly unwarranted assumption that the pathology on the other side will be similar.

Core biopsies in children

Neck lumps are in fact a common paediatric presentation. The incidence of reactive lymphadenopathy due to upper respiratory tract infections is high.[36,37] These children are therefore often observed for several weeks or months, and an open dissection under general anaesthetic may be undertaken if the lymphadenopathy does not resolve. In the rare case of malignant disease or serious infection there has usually been a considerable delay in making the diagnosis.

To date we have performed 21 biopsies in children ranging from 3 months to 16 years of age. Of interest is the fact that 19 of these biopsies have been performed under local anaesthetic with no other sedation required. The youngest patient to undergo a cervical node biopsy without sedation was 2 years of age. For the unsedated child, we have developed a technique which varies slightly from the adult approach.

All unsedated paediatric biopsy patients undergo an initial ultrasound scan which, in addition to defining the lesion and the ease of biopsy, enables the operator, an experienced paediatric ultrasonologist, to make an assessment of the child's poise and composure. There are rare cases where the child is so distressed or restless that it would be futile to attempt biopsy without sedation. If the child appears relaxed and compliant a subsequent booking is made for the biopsy. The parents are given a tube of topical local anaesthetic cream (EMLA cream, Astra Pharmaceuticals Ltd, Herts, UK) and an occlusive dressing and are instructed how and where to apply it at home, an hour before the appointment time. The child is not kept waiting and the biopsy is performed after a top-up injection of local anaesthetic which is usually painless. The biopsy is undertaken while the parent is hugging the child or even with the child sitting on the parent's lap. In our experience the vast majority of children take the procedure in their stride. There has only been 1 case out of the 19 cases attempted so far without sedation where the biopsy had to be abandoned and repeated under sedation.

Complications

In 700 core biopsies we have experienced only 2 complications, both of which occurred early in the series. A patient undergoing a core biopsy of a thyroid nodule experienced a local haemorrhage. Although this stabilised within minutes and did not cause any respiratory compromise she was admitted overnight for analgesia and observation. In a further case the trachea was perforated with the stylet of an 18 SWG needle during the biopsy of a low cervical lymph node. The only symptom was a brief haemoptysis which resolved after a few minutes. The ENT surgeon performed an urgent indirect laryngoscopy and discharged the patient home immediately.

We have not encountered any cases of facial nerve damage. This complication is sought actively by the maxillo-facial and ENT surgeons at outpatient follow-up.

The possibility of tumour seeding has been grossly overstated in relation to percutaneous biopsies. Previous series have admittedly described this complication in relation to FNA and not core biopsies, but no cases were found in two published series,[38,39] and only 12 cases of suspected tumour seeding were identified in a further larger review of several thousand FNAs.[40]

Conclusion

There is no doubt that core biopsy is a safe technique. The adequacy of tissue retrieval is always an enigmatic quality to define. Our rate of successful tissue definition is 93%, far higher than any FNA series when the same criteria are imposed. While we are not proposing that core biopsies should replace cytological diagnosis in all instances, the technique is under-utilised at present and is definitely worth exploring as an adjunct to FNA.

Acknowledgement

The author would like to thank Dr Nick Screaton for his contribution and support in the writing of this section.

References

Fine-needle aspiration

1. Orell SV, Sterrett GF, Walters MNI, Whittaker D. *Manual and Atlas of Fine Needle Aspiration Cytology.* Edinburgh: Churchill Livingstone, 1992; pp 2–21.
2. Layfield L. Fine-needle aspiration of the head and neck. In: Ljung B, ed. *Fine-Needle Aspiration Biopsy. Pathology: State of the Art Reviews.* Philadelphia: Hanley & Belfus, 1996; vol 4, pp 409–438.
3. Gosepath K, Hinni M, Mann W. The state of the art of ultrasonography in the head and neck (editorial). *Ann Otolaryngol Chir Cervicofac* 1994; **111(1):** 1–5.
4. Takes RP, Righi P, Meeuwis CA *et al.* The value of ultrasound with ultrasound-guided fine-needle aspiration biopsy compared to computed tomography in the detection of regional metastases in the clinically negative neck. *Int J Radiat Oncol Biol Phys* 1998; **40(5):** 1027–1032.
5. Righi PD, Kopecky KK, Caldemeyer KS, Ball VA, Weisberger EC, Radpour S. Comparison of ultrasound-fine needle aspiration and computed tomography in patients undergoing elective neck dissection. *Head-Neck* 1997; **19(7):** 604–610.
6. Atula TS, Varpula MJ, Kurki TJ, Klemi PJ, Grenman R. Assessment of cervical lymph node status in head and neck cancer patients: palpation, computed tomography and low field magnetic resonance imaging compared with ultrasound-guided fine-needle aspiration cytology. *Eur J Radiol* 1997; **25(2):** 152–161.
7. van den Brekel MW, Pameijer FA, Koops W, Hilgers FJ, Kroon BB, Balm AJ. Computed tomography for the detection of neck node metastases in melanoma patients. *Eur J Surg Oncol* 1998; **24(1):** 51–54.
8. Takes R, Knegt P, Manni J *et al.* Regional metastasis in head and neck squamous cell carcinoma: revised value of US with US-guided FNAB. *Radiology* 1996; **198:** 819–823.
9. Boland G, Lee M, Mueller P, Mayo-Smith W, Dawson S, Simeone J. Efficacy of sonographically guided biopsy of thyroid masses and cervical lymph nodes. *AJR* 1993; **161:** 1053–1056.
10. Patt B, Schaefer SD, Vuitch F. Role of fine-needle aspiration in the evaluation of neck masses. *Med Clin North Am* 1993; **77:** 611–623.
11. Silverman S, Lee B, Mueller P, Cibas E, Seltzer S. Impact of positive findings at image-guided biopsy of lymphoma on patient care: evaluation of clinical history, needle size, and pathologic findings on biopsy performance. *Radiology* 1994; **190:** 759–764.
12. McIvor N, Freeman J, Salem S, Elden L, Noyek A, Bedard Y. Ultrasonography and ultrasound-guided fine-needle aspiration biopsy of head and neck lesions: a surgical perspective. *Laryngoscope* 1994; **104:** 669–674.
13. Carney AS, Sharp JF, Cozens NJA. Atypically located submandibular gland diagnosed by Doppler ultrasound. *J Laryngol Otol* 1996; **110(12):** 1171–1172.
14. Robinson IA, Cozens NJA. Does a joint ultrasound guided cytology clinic optimise the cytological evaluation of head and neck masses? *Clin Radiol* 1999; **54:** 312–316.
15. van den Brekel MW, Castelijns JA, Snow G. The size of lymph nodes in the neck on sonograms as a radiologic criterion of metastasis: how reliable is it? *Am J Neuroradiol* 1998; **19:** 695–700.
16. Kruyt RH, van Putten WL, Levendag PC, de Boer MF, Oudkerk M. Biopsy of nonpalpable cervical lymph nodes: selection criteria for ultrasound-guided biopsy in patients with head and neck squamous cell carcinoma. *Ultrasound Med Biol* 1996; **22(4):** 413–419.

17. Hamaker R, Moriarty A, Hamaker R. Fine-needle biopsy techniques of aspiration versus capillary in head and neck masses. *Laryngoscope* 1995; **105**: 1311–1314.

18. Mair S, Dunbar F, Becker PJ, DuPlessis W. Fine needle cytology – is aspiration suction necessary? A study of 100 masses in various sites. *Acta Cytol* 1989; **33**: 809–813.

19. Hopper KD, Grenko RT, Fisher AI, TenHave TR. Capillary versus aspiration biopsy: effect of needle size and length on the cytopathological specimen quality. *Cardiovasc Intervent Radiol* 1996; **19(5)**: 341–344.

20. Akhtar S, Ul-Imran H, Faiz U, Reyes L. Efficacy of fine-needle capillary biopsy in the assessment of patients with superficial lymphadenopathy. *Cancer* 1997; **81**: 277–280.

21. Steel B, Schwartz M, Ramzy I. Fine needle aspiration biopsy in the diagnosis of lymphadenopathy in 1,103 patients. Role, limitations and analysis of diagnostic pitfalls. *Acta Cytol* 1995; **39**: 76–81.

22. Savage CA, Hopper KD, Abendroth CS, Hartzel JS, TenHave TR. Fine-needle aspiration biopsy versus fine-needle capillary (nonaspiration) biopsy: in vivo comparison. *Radiology* 1995; **195(3)**: 815–819.

23. Cozens NJA, Robinson IA. To suck or not to suck? That is the question. Is capillary action suitable for fine needle aspiration? (Abstract) Proceedings of BMUS 13th Annual Meeting, 1998. *Eur J Ultrasound* 1998; **8(3)**: S17.

Core biopsy

24. Piromalli D, Martelli G, Del Prato I *et al*. The role of fine needle aspiration in the diagnosis of thyroid nodules; analysis of 795 consecutive cases. *J Surg Oncol* 1992; **50**: 247–250.

25. Miller JM, Hamburger JI, Kini S. Diagnosis of thyroid nodules. Use of fine-needle aspiration and needle biopsy. *JAMA* 1979; **241**: 481–484.

26. Wool MS. Thyroid nodules. The place of fine-needle aspiration biopsy in management. *Postgrad Med* 1993; **94**: 115–122.

27. Caraway NP, Sneige N, Samaan NA. Diagnostic pitfalls in thyroid fine-needle aspiration: a review of 394 cases. *Diagn Cytopathol* 1993; **9**: 345–350.

28. Sanchez RB, van Sonnenberg E, D'Agostino HB *et al*. Ultrasound guided biopsy of non-palpable and difficult to palpate thyroid masses. *J Am Coll Surg* 1994; **178**: 33–37.

29. Robbins KT, van Sonnenberg E, Casola G *et al*. Image-guided needle biopsy of inaccessible head and neck lesions. *Arch Otolaryngol, Head Neck Surg* 1990; **116**: 957–961.

30. Bain GA, Bearcroft PWP, Berman LH, Grant JW. The use of ultrasound-guided cutting-needle biopsy in paediatric neck masses. *Eur Radiol* in press.

31. Bearcroft PWP, Berman LH, Grant J. The use of ultrasound-guided cutting-needle biopsy in the neck. *Clin Radiol* 1995; **50**: 690–695.

32. Ochi K, Ohashi T, Ogino S *et al*. Biopsy of head and neck lesions with a Biopty biopsy instrument. *Nippon Jibiinkoka Gakkai Kaiho* 1992; **95**: 551–555.

33. Betsill WRJ, Hajdu SI. Percutaneous aspiration biopsy of lymph nodes. *Am J Clin Pathol* 1980; **73**: 471–479.

34. Kline TS, Kannan V, Kline IK. Lymphadenopathy and aspiration biopsy cytology: review of 376 superficial nodes. *Cancer* 1984; **54**: 1076–1081.

35. Ramzy I, Rone R, Schultenover SJ *et al*. Lymph node aspiration biopsy: diagnostic reliability and limitations; an analysis of 350 cases. *Diagn Cytopathol* 1985; **1**: 39–45.

36. Slap GB, Brooks JS, Schwartz JS. When to perform biopsies of enlarged peripheral lymph nodes in young patients. *JAMA* 1984; **252**: 1321–1326.

37. Kardos TF, Maygarden SJ, Blumberg AK, Wakley PE, Frable WJ. Fine needle aspiration in the management of children and young adults with peripheral lymphadenopathy. *Cancer* 1989; **63**: 703–707.

38. Engzell V, Eposti PL, Rubio C *et al*. Investigation of tumour spread in connection with aspiration biopsy. *Acta Radiol Ther* 1971; **10**: 385–387.

39. Owen ERTC, Banerjee AK, Prichard AJN *et al*. Role of fine needle aspiration cytology and computed tomography in the diagnosis of parotid swellings. *Br J Surg* 1989; **76**: 1273.

40. Glazer KS, Weger AR, Schmid KW *et al*. Is fine-needle aspiration of tumours harmless? *Lancet* 1989; **1**: 620.

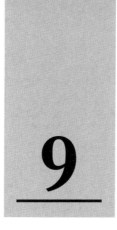

9

CAROTID AND VERTEBRAL ULTRASONOGRAPHY

S S Y Ho, C Metreweli

Anatomy
Examination
Normal ultrasound appearances
Ultrasound appearances of carotid
and vertebral pathology

Introduction

In a chapter concerned with vascular ultrasound of the head and neck it would be pertinent to cover not only the carotid and vertebral arteries but other vessels such as the temporal, ophthalmic and ocular arteries. As space does not permit, this chapter is devoted to the carotids and vertebral, arteries. Furthermore, although there are many diseases that affect the arteries – including dissection, carotid body tumour, arteritis (tuberculosis, Takayasu's), and arteriovenous fistulae – the most common reason for examining the carotids and vertebrals is atheromatosis and its sequelae that lead to cerebral ischaemia. This chapter will therefore concentrate on this aspect of vascular ultrasound.

Ultrasound is non-invasive and more readily available than other techniques – digital subtraction angiography (DSA), computed tomography angiography (CTA) and magnetic resonance angiography (MRA) – and, uniquely, it can visualise the arterial wall itself. All other techniques are currently able to visualise only the lumen and provide very little information about the vessel wall. Ultrasound visualises the wall, the lumen and flowing blood. Doppler or colour flow techniques can provide dynamic information that indicates the haemodynamic effect of any abnormalities discovered. It also provides clues to intracranial disease when the extracranial arteries are normal, even when transcranial Doppler (TCD) or transcranial colour Doppler (TCCD) is unavailable.

Stroke is a significant public health problem, with an incidence of 2.9 per 1000 population in England and Wales[1] with a recurrence rate of between 20% and 50% within 5 years. The estimated survival rate after a second stroke is only 40%.[2] Even with medical therapy, many stroke victims survive with various degrees of residual neurological impairment.

Thromboembolic disease is a major cause of stroke secondary to atherosclerosis, which is the formation of fibrofatty plaques within the intima of the arteries and arterioles. It most frequently affects the carotid bifurcation, carotid siphon, proximal middle cerebral artery, proximal and distal vertebral arteries, and proximal basilar artery.[3] The distribution of cerebrovascular disease is race related. Intracranial atherosclerosis is more common in Chinese, Afrocaribbeans and Japanese while extracranial disease is more prevalent in caucasions.[4]

Atherosclerotic lesions may develop inflammatory changes, cholesterol crystals, necrotic debris, and subintimal haemorrhage. If the plaque ruptures, it may release these materials as emboli and/or cause thrombus formation on the ulcerated surface, thus placing the patient at risk of cerebral thromboembolic disease.[3]

50–60% of patients with transient ischaemic attacks (TIAs) have less than a 50% stenosis on cerebral arteriography.[5] TIAs are followed by stroke within 5 years in 33% of patients, the period of greatest risk being the first two weeks after a TIA.[6] Identification of flow-limiting stenosis is therefore important in assessing the risk of stroke.

The North American Symptomatic Carotid Endarterectomy Trial (NASCET), European Carotid Surgery Trial (ECST) and Asymptomatic Carotid Atherosclerosis Study (ACAS) have clearly demonstrated the benefit of carotid endarterectomy for symptomatic patients with ≥ 70% diameter stenosis.[7–9] These studies emphasize the need for accuracy in the estimation of the degree of carotid stenosis by ultrasound.

It is generally agreed that the prime indication of ultrasound is to identify flow-limiting stenoses, especially high grade stenoses (≥ 70%), in symptomatic patients who are likely to benefit from carotid endarterectomy.

Anatomy

Common carotid artery

The common carotid arteries (CCA) arise from the innominate artery on the right and directly from the arch of the aorta on the left. Each vessel ascends obliquely from behind the sterno-clavicular articulation and divides into the internal carotid artery (ICA) and external carotid artery (ECA), usually at the level of the fourth cervical vertebra.[10] It then widens slightly at the bifurcation into the carotid bulb.

Internal carotid artery

The internal carotid artery (ICA) supplies mainly the anterior part of the brain, the eye, and its appendages.[10] The course of the vessel can be divided into the bulbous, cervical, petrous, cavernous and cerebral portions.[11] Only the first two portions lie extracranially and are readily accessible to sonography.

The first portion of the ICA runs lateral or posterolateral to the ECA in approximately 90% of cases, the angle of divergence depending on age and the length of the vessels.[12] The extracranial portion of the ICA does not give off any branches. The carotid siphon and the ophthalmic artery originate in the cavernous portion.[10] The carotid siphon is a common site for atherosclerotic plaque.[3] The ophthalmic artery is an important anastomotic site between the ICA and ECA to maintain cerebral blood flow when there is extracranial ICA occlusion.[12] The cerebral branches of the ICAs (anterior cerebral artery – ACA, middle cerebral artery – MCA, and posterior communicating artery – PCoA) and vertebral arteries form the circle of Willis.[10] In instances of arterial occlusion in the carotid or vertebrobasilar vessels, this circle functions as a vital collateral pathway through the communicating arteries.[13]

There is normally no branch from the ICA in the cervical region. Occasionally, anomalous branches of the ICA connecting with the occipital or the ascending pharyngeal arteries have been reported and can occasionally be demonstrated extracranially by duplex ultrasound.[14,15]

External carotid artery

The external carotid artery (ECA) plays a vital role in collateral circulation, its branches anastamose with those of the ICA and the vertebral arteries if there is an arterial occlusion of these vessels. The most important collateral pathways are those communicating with the ophthalmic artery and those interconnecting the muscular branches of the occipital and vertebral arteries.[12] The superior thyroid artery, the first branch of the ECA, is readily detected by duplex ultrasound extracranially. It has also been reported arising directly from the CCA.[16] The superficial temporal artery, which is easily palpable in the pre-auricular region, is frequently used, when the sonographer is uncertain of the identity of the vessels, in the tapping manoeuvre for differentiating the ECA from the ICA by noting the disturbance in the ECA Doppler waveform.

Examination

EQUIPMENT

- A high resolution linear transducer

- Duplex or triplex display mode option (real-time grey-scale image ± spectral Doppler analysis ± colour flow imaging)

- Adjustable wall filter, ultrasound beam angle steering, angle correction.

SCANNING PROTOCOL

1 *Patient position*
   - Supine
   - Neck slightly extended
   - Head turned away from the side being examined

2 *Regions of interest*
   - Both CCAs from the origins to the bifurcations
   - Both ICAs and ECAs as cephalad as possible
   - Both vertebral arteries (the proximal and the interforamina segments)

3 *Procedure*
   - Examine the carotid arteries transversely, followed by longitudinal scans
   - Record any plaque formation, its location, extent and morphology
   - Quantify the degree of stenosis, of the ICA in particular, by both grey-scale imaging (i.e. by direct measurement of the luminal reduction) and spectral Doppler analysis (i.e. by predicted percentage reduction by velocity parameters), with the aid of colour flow imaging if necessary
   - Examine the vertebral arteries by duplex sonography
   - Record the findings on a proforma (Appendix 9.1).

Examination technique

CAROTID ARTERIES

Intima–media thickness (IMT)

Evaluation of the vessel wall requires the use of appropriate machine settings. The IMT is defined as the distance between the leading edges of the lumen–intima interface and the media–adventitia interface of the outer wall (Figure 9.1).[17] Measurements should be made on a magnified view to minimise error.

IMT measurements are more reproducible in the CCA than in the ICA or the bifurcation because of its superficial location and relatively straight course.[18]

Luminal diameter and area reduction

Atherosclerotic plaques can be 'concentric' or 'eccentric'. The terms 'circumferential/non-circumferential' or 'symmetric/asymmetric' are also used. The reduction in diameter caused by a concentric plaque will lead to a greater reduction in cross-sectional area than an eccentric plaque (Figure 9.2). An eccentric stenosis could be under- or overestimated by angiography.[12]

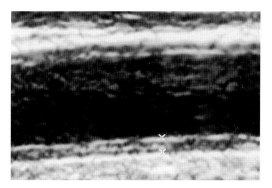

Figure 9.1 – Longitudinal scan of the mid portion of the CCA. The IMT is shown between the two electronic calipers on the far edge of the vessel.

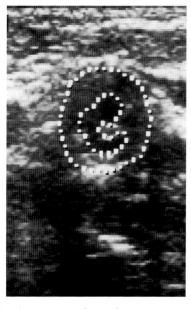

Figure 9.2 – An eccentric plaque showing a severe diameter reduction, but much less severe area reduction.

The measurement of luminal diameter and area reduction should be made on the cross-section of the vessel. Good visualisation of the vessel wall and residual lumen on a true transverse section is crucial because obliquity of the vessel plane will lead to overestimation of the degree of stenosis. Wrongly defined vessel margins may cause erroneous grading of stenosis. In a tight stenosis, where the visualisation of the residual lumen is often poor, colour flow imaging may help in depicting the luminal flow so that measurement of the degree of stenosis is possible, but colour 'blush' over the thickened vessel wall may result in underestimation of the severity of stenosis. In our experience, grading of mild and moderate stenoses is more accurate with direct measurement of the stenosis on a high resolution greyscale image, whereas high grade stenoses are better evaluated by predicted measurement using the Doppler velocity parameters.

Spectral Doppler analysis

When vascular technologists or sonographers perform spectral Doppler analysis to document the degree of stenosis, two velocity parameters are commonly used: peak systolic velocity (PSV) and systolic velocity ratio (SVR).

For velocity measurements, a standardised technique is required to provide accurate results. The velocity measurements for the carotid and vertebral arteries are most easily obtained on longitudinal scans, preferably along a straight segment at least 2 cm away from the bifurcation. Complex flow is present near the bifurcation, leading to inaccurate angle correction. Flow velocity must be angle-corrected, preferably at an angle of 60 degrees or less, as the error resulting from wrong angle correction is unacceptably high at larger angles.[11] Standardisation of angle correction on both sides is important if side-to-side comparison is required.

The size of sample volume may affect the accuracy of peak velocity measurements. Previous authors have suggested a small sample volume is used to obtain the peak systolic velocity at the centre of the vessel, as a larger sample volume introduces spectral broadening.[11] However, a large sample volume that completely encompasses the vessel lumen furnishes more reproducible results; this is advantageous in right-to-left comparison and serial examinations.[12] As a compromise, we recommend that a sample volume of approximately half the size of the vessel lumen placed at the centre of the vessel be interrogated. In a tight stenosis, when the velocity of the stenotic jet is measured, a small sample volume should be used.

The *peak systolic velocity (PSV)* is a reliable and sensitive Doppler velocity parameter. It is considered by some authors to be the single best parameter for quantifying a stenosis and detecting a > 70% stenosis.[19,20] It is the first parameter to become abnormal in arterial disease and will increase with an increasing severity of stenosis.[21] This parameter is dependent upon a group of physiological variables including blood pressure, cardiac output, peripheral resistance and arterial compliance.[22] It also depends on technical variation between different ultrasound machines, transducers and operators.[23,24] Tandem or contralateral obstructive lesions affecting the carotid blood flow are also likely to affect the values of the PSV in the ICA, leading to inaccurate grading of a stenosis.[3,21]

The *systolic velocity ratio (SVR)* is another parameter that is widely employed in conjunction with the PSV to quantify stenoses. It is defined as the ratio of the PSV at the maximal ICA stenosis to the PSV in the normal ipsilateral CCA ($SVR = PSV_{stenosis}/PSV_{normal}\ CcA$).[25] The SVR is claimed to be as good as, or superior to, the PSV in identifying a high grade ($< 70\%$) stenosis. This is because of its physiologically independent nature, its ability to obviate the effects of tandem or contralateral obstructive lesions and the capability of eliminating technical variance.[26]

To obtain the PSV in the normal CCA, the distance from the bifurcation at which CCA velocity is measured should be standardised. This is because the velocity in the CCA is not constant throughout the course of the vessel, but increases with proximity to the aorta.[27] The limitation of this parameter is that it cannot be used if the ipsilateral CCA is diseased. It is a calculated ratio and requires the additional processing of numerical values which may add a small amount of variability to the measurement.[26]

The Doppler velocity parameters mentioned above are generally applied to ICA stenoses.

VELOCITY PARAMETERS
PSV
Reliable and sensitive for detecting and quantifying a high grade stenosis
Dependent upon physiological variables and technical variation
Inaccurate in the presence of tandem or contralateral obstructing lesions
SVR
Good for identifying a high grade stenosis
Physiologically and technically independent
Not affected by tandem or contralateral obstructive lesions
Inapplicable in the presence of a CCA stenosis or occlusion

Differentiation of the extracranial ICA and ECA

The Doppler waveforms of the normal CCA and ICA are of low resistance, in contrast to that of the ECA which is of high resistance (Figure 9.3). Distinction of the ECA from the ICA is not usually a problem with the knowledge of their characteristic waveforms, typical posterolateral location of the ICA with respect to the ECA, and the origin of the superior thyroid artery from the ECA. In difficult cases, digital tapping of the superficial temporal artery may provide a reliable method of identifying the ipsilateral ECA although this manoeuvre will produce waveform oscillations in the ipsilateral ICA and CCA as well. The frequency and strength of responses are, however, more pronounced in the ECA, unaltered by the degree of stenosis in the ECA or in the ICA.[28]

DIFFERENTIATION OF THE EXTRACRANIAL ICA AND ECA
1   There is no branch of the extracranial ICA.
2   The first branch of the ECA – superior thyroid artery – is readily detectable on ultrasound.
3   In 90% of cases, the ICA runs lateral or posterolateral to the ECA.
4   The ICA has a larger calibre than the ECA.
5   The Doppler waveform of the ICA is of low resistance with a high diastolic component while that of the ECA is of high resistance with a low or zero diastolic component.
6   There is prominent disturbance in the ECA Doppler waveform during the 'tapping' manoeuvre of the superficial temporal artery.

Carotid bulb

The complex flow disturbance in the normal carotid bulb may be misinterpreted as an abnormality. This flow pattern is due to the widening of the carotid bulb with disturbance of the laminar flow pattern in the CCA causing flow reversal in the bulb.[29] This area of low shear stress predisposes to the development of atheroma in the carotid bifurcation.[30]

With the aid of colour flow imaging, we are able to demonstrate the complex but characteristic flow pattern in the normal carotid bulb. In early systole, blood

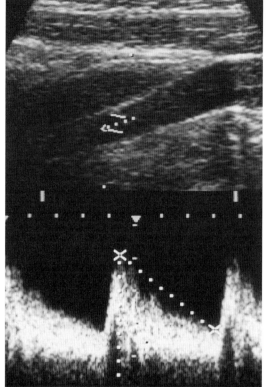

(a)

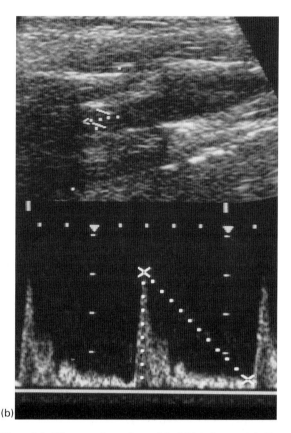

(b)

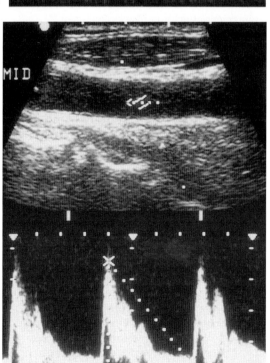

(c)

Figure 9.3 – The spectral waveform of the ICA is characteristically of low resistance with a high diastolic component (a) while that of the ECA is of high resistance with a low diastolic component (b). The waveform of the CCA is usually of low resistance but can also appear as a combination of those of the ICA and ECA (c).

in the carotid bulb is accelerated predominantly in the forward direction. As the peak of systole is approached, a large separation zone with flow reversal develops (A flow separation of separation zone is an area of reversed flow in the fluid layers adjacent to the vessel wall. It occurs at bifurcations, stenoses or at a site of focal dilatation of the vessel lumen). In diastole, the flow in the separate zone becomes virtually static.[29] Flow separation should be seen in every normal individual and absence of this feature should raise the suspicion of plaque formation.

Validation against angiographic technique

Four angiographic measurement techniques are currently used to validate the ultrasound findings: the ECST (E) method,[8] the NASCET (N) method,[7] the

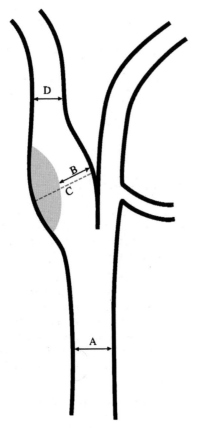

Figure 9.4 – Measurements to be taken at the carotid bifurcation.

and clinician must follow the same protocol and consistently adhere to protocol in follow-up examinations.

Colour flow imaging

The advantages of colour flow imaging are primarily in looking for the residual lumen in a tight stenosis or in assessing an indeterminate total occlusion. It also aids in Doppler spectral sampling at the point of maximal colour shift and angle correction appropriate to the stenotic jet.

Attempts have been made to quantify carotid stenosis by colour Doppler (CDI) or power Doppler imaging (PDI) which is also known as 'colour power angio', and the colour velocity alternatives 'colour velocity power' or 'colour velocity angio'. Several studies have shown that PDI is superior to CDI in depicting the intrastenotic lumen.[34,35] Estimates of stenosis by PDI also correlate better than CDI with arteriography;[34] this may be due to the relative angle independence of PDI, its high sensitivity in depicting the continuity of blood flow and improved intravascular edge definition.[34] PDI is, however, more sensitive to motion artefact, and this is problematic in areas of the vessel with large amounts of tissue motion.[34] The less favourable performance of CDI in characterisation and quantification of severe ICA stenosis, and the visualisation of the residual lumen of a tight stenosis can be significantly improved by administering an intravenous echo-enhancement agent.[36]

common carotid (C) method,[31] and the Carotid Stenosis Index (CSI) method[32] (Figure 9.4).

1   *The (E) method:* stenosis = $(1 - B/C) \times 100\%$

2   *The (N) method:* stenosis = $(1 - B/D) \times 100\%$

3   *The (C) method:* stenosis = $(1 - B/A) \times 100\%$

4   *The Carotid Stenosis Index:* stenosis = $(1 - B/1.2A) \times 100\%$

The (N) method, despite its popularity among radiologists, tends to underestimate the degree of stenosis in the bulb itself.[11] One must therefore be aware that correlation of angiography with ultrasound findings depends on the angiographic stenosis measurement technique, the symmetry of the stenosis, the performance of the ultrasound equipment, and operator-dependent velocimetry. It is hence crucial to have diagnostic criteria and validation processes specific to each individual institution.[33] In addition, the radiologist

CAROTID EXAMINATION

1   The posterolateral approach is used to demonstrate the carotid bifurcation as 90% of ICAs lie lateral or posterolateral to the ECA.

2   Flow velocity must be angle corrected, preferably < 60 degrees.

3   Standardise angle correction on both sides, if side-to-side comparison is required.

4   A large sample volume that completely encompasses the vessel lumen will furnish more reproducible results and is advantageous in right-to-left comparison and repeat examinations.

5   The advantage of colour flow imaging is to speed up the examination by aiding in Doppler spectral sampling at the point of maximal colour shift and angle correction appropriate to the stenotic jet, to depict vessel morphology or diagnose vessel patency.

VERTEBRAL ARTERIES

The vertebral artery (VA) is normally the first and largest branch of the subclavian artery. In about 4% of cases it arises directly from the aortic arch, usually on the left but occasionally on the right. The vessel is divided into four segments (V1 to V4):

1 *V1:* from origin to the point of entry into the transverse foramen of the sixth cervical vertebra

2 *V2:* through the transverse foramina of all the cervical vertebrae

3 *V3:* exiting the first cervical vertebra and running medially in the groove on the upper surface of its posterior arch where muscular branches originate and anastomose with the occipital branches of the ECA

4 *V4:* the intracranial segment from the foramen magnum to its junction with the contralateral vertebral artery to form the basilar artery.[10]

Spectral Doppler analysis usually starts in the V2 region and proceeds downwards to the V1 region and then to its origin. The V3 and V4 regions are not routinely examined if the spectral Doppler waveform is normal in the V2 region.

Examination of the V2 region

With the transducer orientated longitudinally start in the mid cervical region between the trachea and the sternocleidomastoid muscle. Angle the transducer laterally from the CCA and locate the V2 segment posterior to the acoustic shadowing of the transverse processes.

Examination of the V1 region

Trace caudally from V2 to its origin. Compared with the right side, the origin of the left VA is often more difficult to visualise. It is worthy of note that the vertebral vein lying adjacent to the VA can be very pulsatile and mimic an artery. Colour flow imaging will help to differentiate between the two by different colour coding.

The waveform of a normal vertebral artery is of low resistance, similar to that of the CCA but with lower amplitude. The PSV is in the range of 59 ± 17 cm/s and the EDV is 19 ± 8 cm/s.[37] If flow velocity asymmetry is used as a diagnostic criterion for vertebral stenosis or occlusion, the vessel calibre must be taken into account. Discrepancies as small as 1 mm can lead

to asymmetric flow velocities of more than 20 cm/s in PSV. Moreover, a small calibre vertebral artery is relatively frequent. (The vessel is considered hypoplastic when the diameter is smaller than 2 mm.[21]) Other indirect signs of a stenosis may include a decrease in the systolic and, especially, the diastolic velocities, as well as the presence of a high resistivity index over 0.8 in the spectral findings. Often, the contralateral vertebral artery has velocities in the upper limit of the normal range.[38]

Normal ultrasound appearances

The normal carotid arterial wall presents as two distinct echogenic lines separated by an echo-poor zone. The IMT is the distance between the leading edges of the two echogenic lines in the far edge.[18]

The IMT ranges from 0.5 mm to 1.0 mm in healthy adults at all ages;[39] values over 1.0 mm are regarded as abnormal. Detectable atherosclerotic lesions are defined as IMT > 1.2 mm whereas moderate to severe thickening is present when IMT is greater than 2 mm.[40] The wall thickness tends to be greater in the carotid bifurcation than in the CCA, and is larger in men than in women.[39]

The CCA diameter increases with subject size, sex and age.[41] The increase is more marked in males and the CCA diameter is larger in males than in females.[83] The normal dimensions of the carotid arteries are:

1 *CCA:* 6.3 ± 0.9 mm

2 *ICA:* 4.8 ± 0.7 mm

3 *ECA:* 4.1 ± 0.6 mm.[42]

Ultrasound appearances of carotid and vertebral artery pathology

Plaque characterisation

Differences in plaque structure, composition and consistency may account for the relative instability of some atherosclerotic lesions and the resulting clinical outcome.

Plaques are characterised as 'echolucent' or 'echogenic'. The terms 'heterogeneous/homogeneous' or 'soft/dense' are also used. It is proposed that the echolucent (heterogeneous or soft) plaque may con-

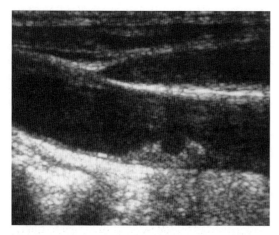

Figure 9.5 – Ultrasound image of a heterogeneous plaque in which the echolucency probably represented intraplaque haemorrhage, lipid deposition or loose proteinaceous deposits.

tain intraplaque haemorrhage (Figure 9.5) which is believed to relate more closely to stroke or transient ischaemic symptoms than the echogenic (homogeneous or hard) fibrous or calcified plaque.[43,44] Apart from intraplaque haemorrhage, the echolucency can also correspond to lipids, cholesterol, or loose proteinaceous deposits.[45] Evidence concerning the correlation of echolucent plaques containing intraplaque haemorrhage with cerebral embolism is conflicting. Several studies have shown that there is no direct correlation between intraplaque haemorrhage and the patient's neurological status and symptoms.[46,47]

Characterisation of the plaque surface morphology is more important, as is shown by the close correlation of ulcerated plaques with subsequent ischaemic events.[48] The reported ability of ultrasound to identify plaque ulceration ranges from less than 30% to more than 90%.[5] Transcutaneous ultrasound, as distinct from intravascular ultrasound, is relatively insensitive in detecting ulcerated surfaces, as is angiography.[47] The ability to detect surface discontinuities in an ulcerated plaque is limited by the lateral resolution of ultrasound imaging instruments. Significant ulcers less than 2 mm can be easily missed.[49] Colour flow imaging may not improve the accuracy of detection because a localised zone of flow reversal, or stagnation of blood flow, which can be seen in the ulcer crater, can also be demonstrated in high grade stenosis.[50] The diagnosis of 'ulcers' is more accurate in plaques when there is less than 50% luminal reduction (Figure 9.6).[12] It becomes unreliable as the degree of stenosis increases.[51]

Intravascular sonography is said to be highly accurate for the diagnosis of plaque ulceration,[52] however the benefit in detecting carotid ulceration must be balanced against the risks of the procedure.

> **PLAQUE CHARACTERISATION**
> Prediction of subsequent stroke by plaque morphology is controversial
> Detection of ulcers in a plaque correlates better with the risk of recurrent cerebral embolism
> Sensitivity for plaque ulceration is poor with transcutaneous ultrasound

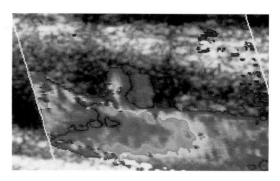

Figure 9.6 – Ultrasound image of an ulcerative plaque. The surface of the plaque is interrupted, with colour flow signals demonstrated in the 'crater'.

Stenoses and occlusions

The establishment of Doppler criteria for grading clinically significant carotid stenoses of 70% or more has become the main objective of most vascular laboratories. These criteria are specific to individual institutions due to the variability of operator technique, ultrasound equipment and validated criteria.[33] The reference values in Table 9.1 show the Doppler criteria for grading carotid stenosis in conformity with NASCET.[53,54] Note that these may not be universally applicable.

Mild ICA stenoses (< 50% diameter reduction)

The velocity proximal or distal to the stenosis is often normal or only slightly increased as the stenosis approaches 50% diameter reduction. The Doppler waveforms of the ipsilateral and contralateral arteries are not affected. The SVR is usually less than 1.5.

Table 9.1 Doppler criteria for grading ICA carotid stenosis

Stenosis (%)	Doppler criteria	
	PSV	*SVR*
< 60	≤ 260 cm/s	< 3.5
≥ 60	> 260 cm/s	> 3.5
≥ 70 (severe)	> 325 cm/s	> 4.0

Data from Moneta *et al.*[53,54]

Moderate ICA stenoses (≥ 50% & < 70% diameter reduction)

The elevation of peak velocity is more marked as the stenosis exceeds 50% diameter reduction. The end-diastolic component of the ipsilateral CCA may be normal or slightly reduced. Eccentric plaques are common, with a clearly defined lumen (if the plaque is not calcified). The ipsilateral and contralateral arteries are not greatly affected. The flow velocity rises sharply as the severity of stenosis increases to 70% diameter reduction.

Severe ICA stenoses (≥ 70% & < 90% diameter reduction)

For a stenosis greater than 70% diameter reduction, both the systolic and diastolic flow velocities remain high (Figure 9.7). Post-stenotic turbulence and aliasing at the stenosis are obvious. The ipsilateral CCA flow may be reduced with low or zero EDV. Collateral flow may be through the ipsilateral ECA or vertebral artery with subsequent increase in flow velocities. Increased contralateral CCA flow may signify cross-over collateralisation.

Subtotal occlusion (≥ 90% diameter reduction)

It has been demonstrated that PSV increases with the severity of stenosis up to 90% diameter reduction and decreases after this point because of flow resistance.[55] It is therefore essential to demonstrate trickle flow (less than 30 cm/s) within the plaque to exclude total occlusion. In the subtotal occlusion, the ipsilateral CCA is invariably affected with low or zero EDV. Concomitant or isolated collateral supply through the ipsilateral ECA and vertebral artery is likely. An increase in contralateral CCA flow, signifying cross-over collateralisation, is common.

Total occlusion

The prevalence of CCA occlusion is relatively low as compared to that of the ICA.[12] Patients with isolated

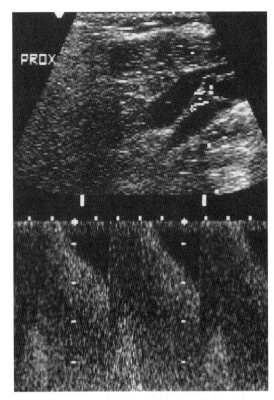

Figure 9.7 – Spectral Doppler of a tight ICA stenosis. Both systolic and diastolic velocities were increased tremendously at the stenosis, exceeding the upper detectable velocity of the equipment.

CCA occlusion may have a better outcome than those with occluded distal vessels. It is therefore very important to document the status of the ICA and ECA in cases of CCA occlusion. Duplex sonography, particularly with colour flow imaging, provides an accurate examination to define the patency of the arteries distal to the carotid bifurcation.

In patients with a potential ICA occlusion it is essential to differentiate a subtotal from a total occlusion, as patients with subtotal ICA occlusion can be managed surgically. A false positive finding of a total occlusion usually results from the limitation of the ultrasound equipment in failing to demonstrate trickle flow within the lumen. Optimal machine settings are hence crucial to minimise misdiagnosis.

In ICA total occlusion, the sonographic findings are similar to those of ICA subtotal occlusion apart from the fact that there is no detectable Doppler signal within the lumen. A typical 'to-and-fro' colour pattern and pre-occlusive 'thump' can be demonstrated proximal to the occluded vessel (Figure 9.8).

In total CCA occlusion, retrograde flow in the ipsilateral ECA may be present in order to supply the cerebral hemisphere of the affected side (Figure 9.9). There may be concomitant or isolated collateral supply from both vertebral arteries or the contralateral CCA.

Isolated total occlusion or stenosis of the ECA

Isolated atheromatous plaque formation in the ECA is uncommon. An ECA occlusion or stenosis is of less clinical importance and it is not interrogated as

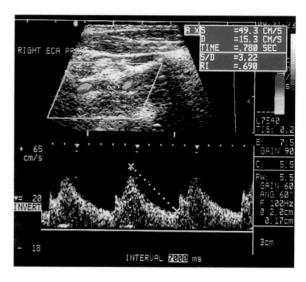

Figure 9.9 – A case of right CCA occlusion with a patent bifurcation. Retrograde flow was demonstrated in the ipsilateral ECA.

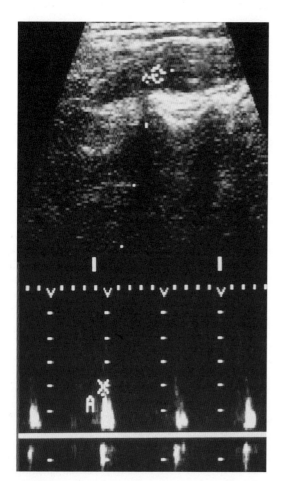

Figure 9.8 – A case of proximal left ICA occlusion. Pre-occlusive 'thumping' was demonstrated just proximal to the occlusion.

intensely as the ICA, but the signs of arterial occlusion such as absence of flow signals within the lumen also apply. The flow velocities are only comparable to those of the ICA in case of severe ECA stenosis, but the flow values are greatly affected by the patency of the ICA.[56]

Stenosis and occlusion of the vertebral arteries

Atherosclerotic lesions of the vertebral arteries commonly occur at the origin of the vertebral artery.[21] Thorough evaluation of the origin is therefore important. Spectral analysis of the V2 segment can give a clue to stenosis or occlusion proximal or distal to it. A high resistive flow pattern without a diastolic flow component, detected in the V2 segment with a normal calibre, is often associated with a distal flow obstruction. A damped waveform with decreased systolic and diastolic components and slow systolic acceleration may be secondary to a severe proximal stenosis (Figure 9.10). The presence of good collaterals may indicate chronic arterial occlusion even though the occluded artery may not be distinct from the surrounding tissue due to intraluminal echogenic thrombus.

A summary of the common duplex findings in carotid stenoses and occlusions is shown in Table 9.2.

Table 9.2 Common duplex findings in carotid stenoses and occlusions

Isolated sites of occlusion	Ipsilateral				Contralateral			
	CCA	ICA	ECA	VA	CCA	ICA	ECA	VA
Total CCA occlusion	Lack of arterial pulsations	Weak antegrade flow	Weak retrograde flow	Normal or increased flow	Increased flow	Increased flow	Normal flow	Normal or increased flow
High-grade carotid bifurcation stenosis	Reduced flow with low or zero EDV	Post-stenotic jet	Post-stenotic jet	Normal or increased flow	Normal flow	Normal flow	Normal flow	Normal flow
Total ICA occlusion	Reduced flow with low or zero EDV	Pre-occlusive 'thump'	Increased flow	Normal or increased flow	Normal flow	Normal flow	Normal flow	Normal flow
Subtotal ICA ≥ 90% stenosis	Reduced flow with low or zero EDV	Trickle flow < 30 cm/s	Increased flow	Normal or increased flow	Normal flow	Normal flow	Normal flow	Normal flow
Severe ICA ≥ 70% stenosis	Reduced or normal flow	Markedly elevated flow velocities	Increased or normal flow	Increased or normal flow	Normal flow	Normal flow	Normal flow	Normal flow
Moderate ICA ≥ 50% stenosis	Normal flow	Moderately elevated flow velocities	Normal flow	Normal flow	Normal flow	Normal flow	Normal flow	Normal flow
Mild ICA < 50% stenosis	Normal flow	Mildly elevated flow velocities	Normal flow	Normal flow	Normal flow	Normal flow	Normal flow	Normal flow

Follow-up endarterectomy

One of the complications seen in post-endarterectomy patients is re-stenosis due to myointimal hyperplasia. The reported incidence of symptomatic recurrent stenosis ranges from 0% to 8.2%, with an asymptomatic recurrence rate of between 1.3 and 37%.[57] In view of the low re-stenosis incidence and the relatively high incidence of asymptomatic re-stenosis, follow-up scans should be limited to patients with specific indications, e.g. anastomotic leak, arterial re-stenosis or occlusion.

Shortly after operation, the carotid wall at the endarterectomy site loses the double line echo as seen in the normal carotid artery. The double line echo then reappears approximately three months postoperatively. This represents a marker of arterial wall healing and signifies that the patient is less likely to develop re-stenosis due to myointimal hyperplasia.[58]

Postoperatively, the proximal 'shelf' at the point of transection can be used as the landmark for assessing the myointimal thickening. The myointimal hyperplasia response is nearly always complete within the first two years; any changes that take place after two years post endarterectomy should be ascribed to atherosclerosis.[11]

Subclavian steal

Subclavian steal syndrome is caused by an occlusion of the proximal subclavian or innominate artery leading to reversal of blood flow in the vertebral artery because blood is 'stolen' from the ipsilateral vertebral artery to supply the hypoperfused arm.[59] As it takes time for the occlusion to develop from stenosis, transitional forms of antegrade to complete retrograde vertebral flow may be encountered. These can be demonstrated with spectral analysis (Figure 9.11). In mild or moderate

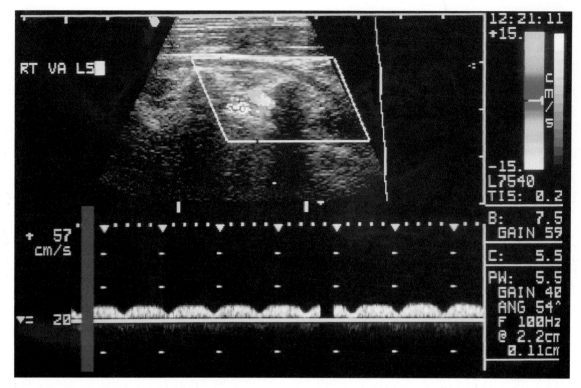

Figure 9.10 – The Doppler spectrum showed a very damped arterial waveform in the V2 region. This finding is highly suggestive of a severe stenosis in the proximal vertebral artery.

stenosis of the subclavian artery, only systolic deceleration of the vertebral flow is observed. As the stenosis progresses, alternating vertebral flow may be detected. If the subclavian artery is totally occluded by atherosclerotic plaque, complete reversal of flow in the ipsilateral vertebral artery will be apparent.[12] The latter two forms of subclavian steal phenomena have been reported to be associated with the occurrence of vertebrobasilar symptoms.[60]

Subclavian steal can be accurately diagnosed by colour duplex sonography, both extracranially and transcranially. This non-invasive technique is sensitive and more superior than angiography as it can demonstrate abnormal transient basilar or vertebral flow in response to an arm compression test, whereas routine angiography may fail to document this condition, presumably due to the forced injection of contrast media which conceals less severe steal at rest.[61]

Arteriovenous fistulas (AVF)

Most arteriovenous fistulas in the neck are acquired secondary to penetrating injuries or as a complication of cannulation of the internal jugular vein. A large AVF is easily diagnosed by duplex ultrasound with the demonstration of abnormal communication between the artery and vein (Figure 9.12). At the communication, the feeding artery is usually of low resistance with a high diastolic component (Figure 9.13a). Turbulence and perivascular colour flow artefacts are common (Figure 9.13b). The arterial Doppler signal distal to the communicating canal may be normal. With large fistulas, 'arterialisation' of the venous signal may occur (Figure 9.13c).

SONOGRAPHIC FINDINGS OF AN ARTERIOVENOUS FISTULA
Abnormal communication between the artery and vein
Low resistance flow with a high diastolic component in the feeding artery
Turbulence and perivascular colour flow artefacts in the arteriovenous fistula
'Arterialisation' of venous signal

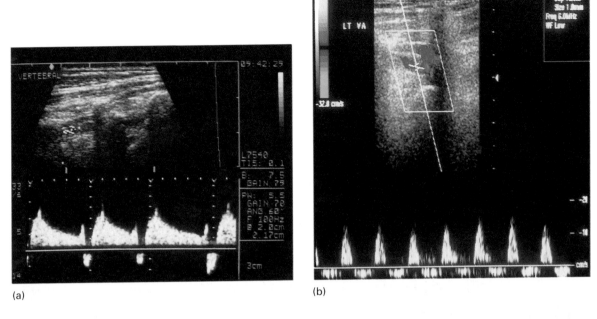

(a)

(b)

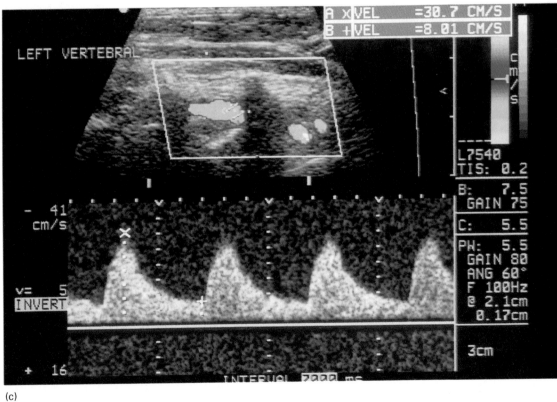

(c)

Figure 9.11 – Different forms of subclavian steal. (a) Systolic deceleration of the vertebral flow. (b) Alternating vertebral flow. (c) Complete flow reversal in the vertebral artery (note the colour coding for flow direction).

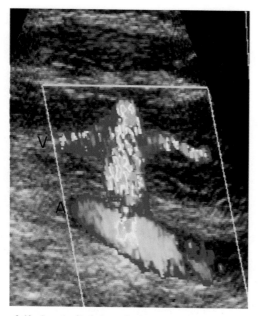

Figure 9.12 – Longitudinal view of an iatrogenic arteriovenous fistula in the neck of a patient. Abnormal communication between the artery and vein with turbulent flow evident.

Carotid and vertebral dissection

Dissection of the large extracranial arteries, commonly the ICA or vertebral artery, is a frequent cause of stroke in children and young adults. Usually, the dissection separates the intima from the media, causing arterial embolism or occlusion with subsequent TIAs or cerebral infarction. Trauma, mild or severe, often accounts for the dissection. Spontaneous dissection can occur in atheromatous lesions, fibromuscular dysplasia, arteritis or in association with a vertebral artery anomaly.[62,63] Patients may present with Horner's syndrome, self-audible bruit, neck pain or transient mono-ocular blindness.[64] Colour duplex sonography is useful for early diagnosis of extracranial neck artery dissection and for follow-up examinations.

The most common site of vertebral dissection is in the distal V1 segment, before it enters the transverse foramen of the sixth cervical vertebra, where the artery is believed to be under greatest mechanical stress.[65]

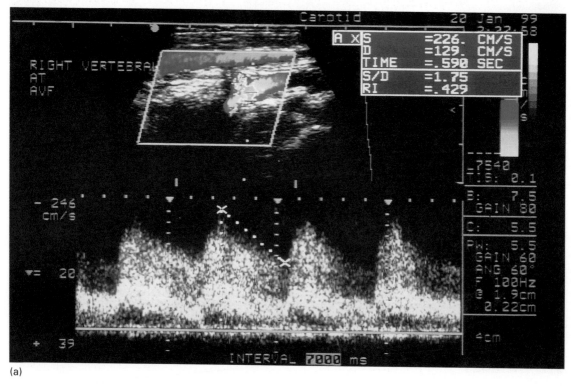

(a)

Figure 9.13 – Longitudinal view of the neck illustrating an iatrogenic arteriovenous fistula of the vertebral artery and vein. At the AVF, there was a high diastolic component in the Doppler waveform (a). *Continued*

Anomalous dual origin or fenestration of the vertebral artery is infrequently reported. It is usually on the left but occasionally on the right or less commonly bilaterally.[66] This anomaly may mimic dissection or predispose to spontaneous dissection.

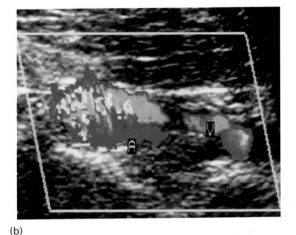

(b)

The typical ultrasound findings of a dissection are:

- dissecting membrane with a true and false lumen
- localised increase in arterial diameter
- tapering stenosis with distal occlusion.[21]

On Doppler, a highly typical, but not pathognomonic signal with systolic forward-and-backward flow may be demonstrated. This is called the 'slosh' phenomenon (Figure 9.14). If the dissection progresses, the slosh phenomenon shifts cranially, and the lumen reopens. In contrast to carotid dissection, the 'slosh' phenomenon is less frequent in vertebral dissection, accounting for about one third of the cases.[67] Spontaneous recanalisation may occur, usually after an average of 4–6 weeks later. During this process, various stenotic signs may be detected with Doppler sonography. These may change daily. Only rarely does the blood vessel remain completely occluded.[66] Treatment involves heparinisation and observation as recanalisation is common.

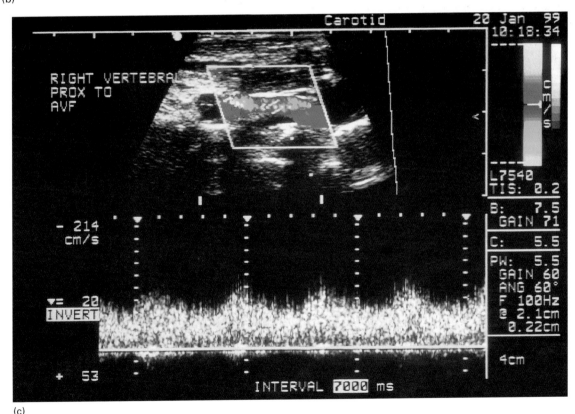

(c)

Figure 9.13 – *Continued* Note the perivascular flow artefact at the communication (b) and 'arterialisation' of the vertebral venous signals (c).

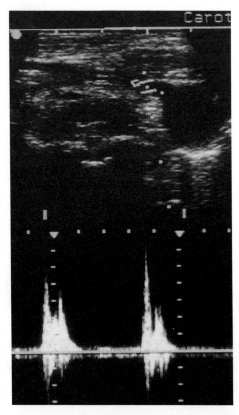

Figure 9.14 – The Doppler spectrum of a vertebral artery showing a 'slosh' phenomenon with synchronous 'to-and-fro' components in the systole. This phenomenon may suggest arterial occlusion secondary to dissection.

SONOGRAPHIC FINDINGS OF A CAROTID/VERTEBRAL DISSECTION
Dissecting membrane with a true and false lumen
Localised increase in arterial diameter
Tapering stenosis with distal occlusion
Systolic 'to-and-fro' flow proximal to the dissection – the 'slosh' phenomenon.

Conclusions

The application of colour duplex ultrasonography in cerebrovascular disease plays an integral part in the diagnostic characterisation of plaque morphology, quantification of stenosis and detection of vascular abnormalities.

Appendix 9.1

Cerebrovascular Arterial Doppler Ultrasound Report
Ultrasound Vascular Laboratory

Patient's Name:	
Sex/Age:	Scan No:
Referral:	
ID No:	Date:

Clinical Hx:

Spectral Doppler and TCCD Findings

Velocity (cm/s)	R Systolic	R Diastolic	L Systolic	L Diastolic
CCA				
ICA				
ECA				
VA				
Stenosis (maximal)				

TCCD (cm/s)	R (S)	R (D)	L (S)	L (D)
MCA				
ACA				
PCA (P1)				
PCA (P2)				
V4				
Basilar				

Findings on the Maximal Stenosis

	R		L	
Site	–		–	
Systolic Ratio	–		–	
Stenosis	Diameter	Area	Diameter	Area
Predicted %	–	–	–	–
Measured %	–	–	–	–

R   L

Comments:

Radiologist	Vascular Technologist	Date

References

1. Department of Health. *Stroke: an Epidemiological Overview; the Health of the Nation.* London: Her Majesty's Stationery Office, 1994.

2. National Institutes of Health. *Arteriosclerosis 1981. Report of the Working Group on Arteriosclerosis of the National Heart, Lung and Blood Institute,* vol 2. Washington DC: NIH, 1981; publication no 82-2035.

3. Naidich TP, Alberto MR. Neurovascular imaging. *Radiol Clin North Am* 1995; **33(1):** 115–166.

4. Feldmann E, Daneault N, Kwan E, Ho KJ, Pessin MS, Langenberg P, Caplan LR. Chinese–white differences in the distribution of occlusive cerebrovascular disease. *Neurology* 1990; **40:** 1541–1545.

5. Bluth EI. Evaluation and characterization of carotid plaque. *Semin Ultrasound CT MR* 1997; **18(1):** 57–65.

6. Gautier JC, Juillard JBE, Lovon PHL *et al.* The interval between transient ischemic attacks and cerebral infarction. *Stroke* 1987; **18:** 298.

7. North American Symptomatic Carotid Endarterectomy Trial Collaborators. Beneficial effect of carotid endarterectomy in symptomatic patients with high-grade carotid stenosis. *N Engl J Med* 1991; **325:** 445–453.

8. European Carotid Surgery Trialists Collaborative Group. MRC European carotid surgery trial: interim results for symptomatic patients with severe (70–99%) or with mild (0–29%) carotid stenosis. *Lancet* 1991; **337:** 1235–1243.

9. Executive Committee for the Asymptomatic Carotid Atherosclerosis Study. Endarterectomy for asymptomatic carotid artery stenosis. *JAMA* 1995; **273:** 1421–1428.

10. Gray H. *Gray's Anatomy – Descriptive and Surgical. The Illustrated Running Press Edition of the American Classic.* Philadelphia: Running Press, 1974.

11. Strandness DE, Jr. *Duplex Scanning in Vascular Disorders,* 2nd edn. New York: Raven Press, 1993; pp 113–157.

12. Von Reutern GM, von Büdingen HJ. *Ultrasound Diagnosis of Cerebrovascular Disease – Doppler Sonography of the Extra- and Intracranial Arteries, Duplex Scanning.* Stuttgart: Thieme, 1993.

13. Diethrich E. Normal cerebrovascular anatomy and collateral pathways. In: Zwiebel WJ (ed) *Introduction to Vascular Ultrasonography,* 3rd edn. Philadelphia: WB Saunders, 1992; pp 87–94.

14. Verbeeck N, Hammer F, Goffette P, Mathurin P. Saccular aneurysm of the external jugular vein, an unusual cause of neck swelling. *J Belge Radiol* 1997; **80(2):** 63–64.

15. Bowen JC, Garcia M, Garrard CL, Mankin CJ, Fluke MM. Anomalous branch of the internal carotid artery maintains patency distal to a complete occlusion diagnosed by duplex scan. *J Vasc Surg* 1997; **26(1):** 164–167.

16. Akyol MU, Koc C, Ozcan M, Ozdem C. Superior thyroid artery arising from the common carotid artery. *Otolaryngol Head Neck Surg* 1997; **116**(6pt1): 701.

17. Nosoe C, Engel U, Karstrup S. The aortic wall. An in vitro study of the double-line pattern in high-resolution US. *Radiology* 1990; **175:** 387–390.

18. Kanters SDJM, Algra A, van Leeuwen MS, Banga JD. Reproducibility of in vivo carotid intima–media thickness measurements – a review. *Stroke* 1997; **28(3):** 665–671.

19. Hunink MGM, Polak JF, Barlan MM, O'Leary D. Detection and quantification of carotid artery stenosis: efficacy of various doppler velocity parameters. *AJR* 1993; **160:** 619–625.

20. Schwartz SW, Chambless LE, Baker WH, Broderick JP, Howard G. Consistency of doppler parameters in predicting arteriographically confirmed carotid stenosis. *Stroke* 1997; **28(2):** 343–347.

21. Zwiebel WJ. *Introduction to Vascular Ultrasonography,* 3rd edn. Philadelphia: WB Saunders, 1992.

22. Kohler T, Langlois Y, Roederer GO *et al.* Sources of variability in carotid duplex examination. *Ultrasound Med Biol* 1985; **11:** 571–576.

23. Hoskins PR. Accuracy of maximum velocity estimates made using doppler ultrasound systems. *BJR* 1996; **69:** 172–177.

24. Ranke C, Trappe HJ. Blood flow velocity measurements for carotid stenosis estimation: interobserver variation and interequipment variability. *Vasa* 1997; **26(3):** 210–214.

25. Keagy BA, Pharr WF, Thomas D, Bowles DE. Evaluation of the peak frequency ratio (PRF) measurement in the detection of internal carotid artery stenosis. *J Clin Ultrasound* 1982; **10:** 109–112.

26. Zwiebel WJ. New doppler parameters for carotid stenosis. *Semin Ultrasound CT MR* 1997; **18(1):** 66–71.

27. Meyer JI, Khalil RM, Obuchowski NA, Baus LK. Common carotid artery: variability of doppler US velocity measurements. *Radiology* 1997; **204:** 339–341.

28. Kliewer MA, Freed KS, Hertzberg BS *et al.* Temporal artery tap: usefulness and limitations in carotid sonography. *Radiology* 1996; **201(2):** 481–484.

29. Ku DN, Giddens DP, Phillips DJ, Strandness DE. Hemodynamics of the normal human carotid bifurcation: in vitro and in vivo studies. *Ultrasound Med Biol* 1985; **11(1):** 13–26.

30. Lee D, Chiu JJ. Intimal thickening under shear in a carotid bifurcation – a numerical study. *J Biomechanics* 1996; **29(1):** 1–11.

31. Alexandrov AV, Brodie DS, McLean A, Hamilton P, Murphy J, Burns PN. Correlation of peak systolic velocity and angiographic measurement of carotid stenosis revisited. *Stroke* 1997; **28(2):** 339–342.

32. Bladin CF, Alexandrova NA, Murphy J, Alexandrova AV, Maggisano R, Norris JW. The clinical value of methods to measure carotid stenosis. *Int Angiol* 1996; **15(4):** 295–299.

33. Kuntz KM, Polak JF, Whittemore AD, Skillman JJ, Kent KC. Duplex ultrasound criteria for the identification of carotid stenosis should be laboratory specific. *Stroke* 1977; **28(3):** 597–602.

34. Griewing B, Morgenstern C, Driesner F, Kallwellis G, Walker ML, Kessler C. Cerebrovascular disease assessed by color-flow and power doppler ultrasonography. Comparison with digital subtraction angiography in internal carotid artery stenosis. *Stroke* 1996; **27(1):** 95–100.

35. Steinke W, Ries S, Artemis N, Schwartx A, Hennerici M. Power doppler imaging of carotid artery stenosis – comparison

with color doppler flow imaging and angiography. *Stroke* 1997; **28(10):** 1981–1987.

36. Sitzer M, Rose G, Furst G, Siebler M, Steinmetz H. Characteristics and clinical value of an intravenous echo-enhancement agent in evaluation of high-grade internal carotid stenosis. *J Neuroimaging* 1997; **7**(Suppl 1): S22–S25.

37. Pfadenhauer K, Muller H. Color-coded duplex ultrasound of the vertebral artery: normal findings and pathologic findings in obstruction of the vertebral artery and remaining cerebral arteries. *Ultraschall Med* 1995; **16(5):** 228–233.

38. Bartels E. Vertebral sonography. In: Tegeler CH, Babikian VL, Gomez CR (eds) *Neurosonology*. St Louis: Mosby, 1996; pp 83–100.

39. Howard G, Sharrett R, Heiss G, Evans GW, Chambless LE, Riley WA, Burke GL. Carotid artery intimal-medial thickness distribution in general populations as evaluated by B-mode ultrasound. *Stroke* 1993; **24(9):** 1297–1304.

40. Salonen R, Seppanen K, Rauramaa R, Salonen JT. Prevalence of carotid atherosclerosis and serum cholesterol levels in Eastern Finland. *Arteriosclerosis* 1988; **8:** 788–792.

41. Polak JF, Kronmal RA, Tell GS *et al*. Compensatory increase in common carotid artery diameter. Relation to blood pressure and artery intima-media thickness in older adults. Cardiovascular health study. *Stroke* 1996; **27(11):** 2012–2015.

42. Schöning M, Walter J, Scheel P. Estimation of cerebral blood flow through color duplex sonography of the carotid and vertebral arteries in healthy adults. *Stroke* 1994; **25(1):** 17–22.

43. Cave EM, Pugh ND, Wison RJ *et al*. Carotid artery duplex scanning: does plaque echogenicity correlate with patient symptoms? *Eur J Vasc Surg* 1995; **10:** 77–81.

44. Iannuzi A, Wilcosky T, Mercuri M *et al*. Ultrasonographic correlates of carotid atherosclerosis in transient ischemic attacks and stroke. *Stroke* 1995; **26:** 614–619.

45. Bock RW, Lusby RJ. Carotid plaque morphology and interpretation of the echolucent lesion. In: Labs K, Jager K, Fitzgerald D *et al* (eds) *Diagnostic Vascular Ultrasound*. London: Edward Arnold, 1992; pp 225–235.

46. Agapitos E, Kavantzas N, Bakouris M *et al*. Estimation of the percentage of carotid atheromatous plaque components and investigation of a probable correlation with the neurologic status of the patients. *Gen Diagn Pathol* 1996; **142(2):** 105–108.

47. Hatsukami TS, Ferguson MS, Beach KW *et al*. Carotid plaque morphology and clinical events. *Stroke* 1997; **28(1):** 95–100.

48. Eliasziw M, Streifler JY, Fox AJ, Hachinski VC, Ferguson GG, Barnett HJ. Significance of plaque ulceration in symptomatic patients within high-grade carotid stenosis. *Stroke* 1994; **25:** 304–308.

49. Hennerici M, Reifschneider G, Trockel U, Aulich A. Detection of early atherosclerotic lesions by duplex scanning of the carotid artery. *J Clin Ultrasound* 1984; **12:** 455–464.

50. Furst H, Hartl WH, Jansen I *et al*. Color-flow doppler sonography in the identification of ulcerative plaques in patients with high-grade carotid artery stenosis. *AJNR* 1992; **13:** 1581–1587.

51. Sitzer M, Muller W, Rademacher J, Siebler M, Hort W, Kniemeyer HW, Steinmetz H. Color-flow doppler-assisted duplex imaging fails to detect ulcerations in high-grade internal carotid artery stenosis. *J Vasc Surg* 1996; **23(3):** 461–465.

52. Miskolczi L, Guterman LR, Flaherty JD, Hopkins LN. Depiction of carotid plaque ulceration and other plaque-related disorders by intravascular sonography: a flow chamber study. *AJNR* 1996; **17(10):** 1881–1890.

53. Moneta GL, Edwards JM, Chitwood RW, Taylor LM Jr, Lee RW, Cummings CA, Porter JM. Correlation of North American Symptomatic Carotid Endarterectomy Trial (NASCET) angiographic definition of 70% to 99% internal carotid artery stenosis with duplex scanning. *J Vasc Surg* 1993; **17:** 152–159.

54. Moneta GL, Edwards JM, Papanicolaou G *et al*. Screening for asymptomatic internal carotid artery stenosis: Duplex criteria for discriminating 60% to 99% stenosis. *J Vasc Surg* 1995; **21:** 989–994.

55. Bluth EI, Stavros AT, Marich KW, Wetzner SM, Aufichtig D, Baker JD. Carotid duplex sonography: a multicenter recommendation for standardized imaging and Doppler criteria. *Radiographics* 1988; **8:** 487–506.

56. Paivansalo MJ, Siniluoto TM, Tikkakoski TA, Myllyla V, Suramo IJ. Duplex US of the external carotid artery. *Acta Radiol* 1996; **37(1):** 41–45.

57. Lattimer CR, Burnand KG. Recurrent carotid stenosis after carotid endarterectomy. *Br J Surg* 1997; **84(9):** 1206–1219.

58. Caps MT, Hatsukami TS, Primozich JF, Bergelin RO, Strandness DE Jr. A clinical marker for arterial wall healing: the double line. *J Vasc Surg* 1996; **23(1):** 87–93.

59. Reivich M, Hollins HE, Roberts B, Toole JF. Reversal of blood flow through the vertebral artery and its effects on cerebral circulation. *N Engl J Med* 1961; **265:** 878–885.

60. Thomassen L, Aarli JA. Subclavian steal phenomenon. Clinical and hemodynamic aspects. *Acta Neurol Scand* 1994; **90(4):** 241–244.

61. Yip PK, Liu HM, Hwang BS, Chen RC. Subclavian steal phenomenon: a correlation between duplex sonographic and angiographic findings. *Neuroradiology* 1992; **34(4):** 279–282.

62. Stahmer SA, Raps EC, Mines DI. Carotid and vertebral artery dissections. *Emerg Med Clin North Am* 1997; **15(3):** 677–698.

63. Kimura K, Yonemitsu M, Hashimoto Y, Uchino M. Spontaneous dissection associated with proximal vertebral artery anomaly. *Intern Med* 1997; **36(11):** 834–836.

64. Kistler JP, Ropper AH, Martin JB. Cerebrovascular disease. In: Braunwald E, Isselbacher KJ, Petersdorf RG, Wilson JD, Martin JB, Fauci AS (eds) *Harrison's Principles of Internal Medicine,* 7th edn. New York: McGraw-Hill, 1987; vol 2, pp 1930–1960.

65. Friedman DP, Flanders AE. Unusual dissection of the proximal vertebral artery: description of three cases. *AJNR* 1992; **13:** 283–286.

66. Takasato Y, Hayashi H, Kobayashi T *et al*. Duplicated origin of right vertebral artery with rudimentary and accessory left vertebral arteries. *Neuroradiology* 1992; **34:** 287–289.

67. Hennerici M, Neuerbury-Heusler D. *Vascular Diagnosis With Ultrasound – Clinical References With Case Studies*. Thieme: New York, 1998; pp 25–88.

INDEX

liposarcoma 101
lymph nodes 72, 75, 101, 124
masses 87, 100–1
nerve sheath tumour 101
third branchial cleft cyst 101
postoperative imaging 127
pre-auricular sinus 95–6
pre-epiglottic space 15, 108, 109, 114
    supraglottic tumour spread 111,
        116
prelaryngeal nodes 73
pre-operative investigations 121–7
    clinical examination 121, 122
    fine-needle aspiration biopsy
        (FNAB) 122
    lymph nodes assessment 122–7
prethyroid nodes 73
pretracheal nodes 73
'pull up surgery' 102

Q

quality of life 127

R

radical neck dissection 124–5
    modified procedure 125
radiotherapy-associated salivary gland
    inflammation 26
ranula 32, 88
recurrent laryngeal nerve palsy 62
recurrent tumour 127
renal cell carcinoma 51
retromandibular vein 9, 11, 20, 21, 70
retropharyngeal nodes 74, 75

S

salivary gland 19–32
    abscess 23, 24, 25
    anatomy 19–21
    calculi 22–4
    core biopsy 142
    cystic mass 32
    examination technique 21–2
    fatty infiltraion 24
    hypertrophy 24

inflammatory disease
    acute 24
    chronic 25–6
    trauma 26
    tumours 26–31, 122
        benign 27–9
        malignant 29–31
    viral infection 24–5
sarcoidosis 26
scalene muscle 13
scalenus anterior muscle 13, 15
schwannoma 98–9
selective neck dissection 125–6
sialadenitis 24
sialectasis 23
sialocele 23
sialolithiasis 22–4
Sjögren's syndrome 25–6
spaces of neck 6
specimen handling 134, 138
spectral Doppler analysis
    carotid arteries 149–50
    subclavian steal 157–8
    vertebral arteries 153
spinal accessory chain (posterior
    triangle lymph nodes) 13, 14, 72,
    75
spinal accessory nerve (XI) 13, 14, 72
    radical neck dissection 125
splenius capitis muscle 13
squamous cell carcinoma
    extranodal spread 122, 123
    lymph nodes metastases 122
        detection 82
        levels 74
        outcome 127
        staging 82
Stensen's duct 20
    trauma 26
sternohyoid muscle 108
sternomastoid muscle 5–6, 13, 14, 15,
    72
    haemangiomas 96
    radical neck dissection 125
sternothyroid muscle 107, 108
strap muscles 15, 16, 107, 108, 109
    thyroid nodule evaluation 42
stroke 147, 154, 160

subclavian artery 13
    stenosis 157, 158
subclavian steal 157–8, 159
subclavian triangle 12
subclavian vein 15
sublingual gland 7
    mucocele (ranula) 32
    tumours 26, 29
sublingual space 7, 8, 20
    contents 20–1
submandibular duct 7, 8
    calculi 23
submandibular gland 8, 9, 69
    calculi 22, 23
    tumours 26, 29, 30
    venous landmarks 9
submandibular region 5, 7, 8, 10,
    20–1
    anatomical aspects 8–9
    congenital cystic lesions 91–2
    contents of space 20
    cystic hygroma 92–3
    lymph nodes 69–70, 74, 89
        criteria of malignancy 76
    lymphatic malformations 92
    masses 87, 89–94
    thyroglossal duct cyst 93–4
submental region 5, 15
    anatomical aspects 7–8
    congenital cystic lesions 88–9
    lymph nodes 7, 68–9, 74, 87
        criteria of malignancy 76
    masses 87–9
superficial venous anatomy 9
superior mediastinal lymph nodes 75
superior thyroid artery 38
superior thyroid vein 38
suppurative sialadenitis, acute 24
suppurative thyroiditis, acute 57
supraclavicular region 5
    anatomical aspects 14–15
supra-omohyoid neck dissection 125
symphysis mentis 7
syphilis 24
syringe holders 133–4
syringes 133, 134
systolic velocity ratio (SVR) 149,
    150